HERBAL BASICS

Heal Your Family Naturally From The Outside In!

By: Arianna Mojica

"Doctors pour drugs of which they know little, to cure diseases of which they know less, into human beings of whom they know nothing."

~ Voltaire

HERBAL BASICS
Heal Your Family Naturally From The Outside In!

Copyright 2015 Arianna Mojica
PO Box 52 , Mackville, KY 40040
Email: mmspublishinggroup@yahoo.com

LIMIT OF LIABILITY/DISCLAIMER: The expressions contained herein may not be suitable for every situation. This work is sold with the understanding that the publisher and author are not engaged in rendering medical or other professional advice. Readers should be aware that any websites listed in this work may have changed or disappeared between the time this work was written and when it is actually read. The information being shared in this book is not meant to diagnose, cure, treat, or prevent any disease. This information has not been evaluated by the Food and Drug Administration (FDA). The reader should be aware that herbs contain natural medicinal properties and should be treated with respect. This book is not intended as a medical reference book, but merely as a source of information written based on the author's life experience and research. Do not take any herbal remedies if you are undergoing any course of medical treatment without seeking professional advice. Before trying herbal remedies, the reader is advised to sample a small quantity to establish whether there is any adverse or allergic reaction. The reader is advised not to attempt self-treatment for serious long-term problems, during pregnancy or for children without consulting a qualified medicinal herbalist. Neither the author nor the publisher can be held responsible for any adverse reactions to the formulations, suggestions, and instructions contained herein. The use of any herb or derivative is entirely at the reader's own discretion and risk. Special care should be taken by pregnant or lactating women, when handling herbs. Keep all herbs out of reach of children and pets.

Printed in the United States
Library of Congress Cataloging-in-Publication Data
Mojica, Arianna, Copyright 2015
Herbal Basics – heal your family naturally from the outside in!
ISBN **978-0-578-15621-7**

Dedication:

To my beautiful children, Mikaelah and Malakai. Thank you for never failing to inspire me to be a better mother, friend, and human being. May your free spirits continue to soar, may you both continue to live your purpose, loving life, nature, and learning, so that you may leave this earth better than how you found it. Remember... I will always love, support and guide you, in this existence and beyond. I wish you enough.

To Nanya, my loving husband and partner; thank you for being my biggest supporter and most gentle critic. Thank you for always supporting my creativity and for trusting my womanly instincts to dream bigger dreams for our family. To this day, I am still grateful that the universe heard my cries for you.

HERBAL BASICS

Heal Your Family Naturally

From The Outside In!

By: Arianna Mojica

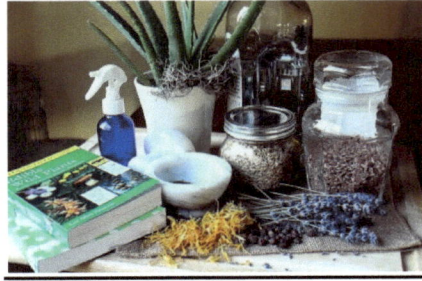

Table of Contents

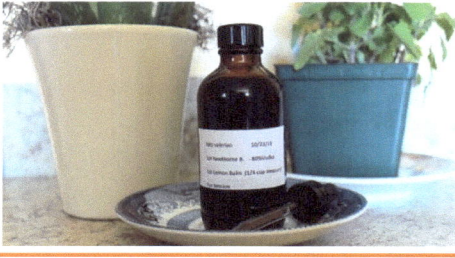

Chapter 1
Back to Basics

If you are reading this book, it is a good indication that you value your health and the health of your family. I honor you for allowing me into your space and for taking such an active role in your wellness.

As most of you are aware, the prescribing of herbs and diagnosing of dis-ease is "against the law" in the U.S.A, unless one holds a current medical degree and license (i.e., pays a fee). For the record, I do not claim to be a medical practitioner. However, I strongly believe it is our natural right to learn about alternative methods in order to counter the aggressive allopathic system that is being pushed so heavily upon us. To that end, it has become my passion and life's purpose to share what has been extremely valuable to our family, as we strive to live a healthier and more balanced life. I will that as you read my expressions, you are inspired to do the same.

It is time we go back to basics. Herbal medicine is the oldest form of medicine known to man. It has been used successfully by every ancient civilization on the face of the earth, yet those that stand to gain the most from its absence in our society are aggressively pushing it into extinction. This is obvious to see when we consider the fact that herbal and holistic medicine is now looked upon with great skepticism - as a taboo even - and is routinely discredited by the "licensed professionals" as quackery.

It might come as a surprise to know that before pharmacies and drug stores where invented, there were apothecaries that dispensed herbal remedies that often functioned the same way pharmacists and doctors do today. Their skills with herbs made them

Allopathic medicine deals with body parts. We are much more complex than the sum of our parts. In sharp contrast, holistic healing involves the whole YOU...mind, body, and spirit!

reliable resources for people seeking natural healing from any ailment. A lot has changed since the days of apothecaries, and it is worth noting that it was only when herbal medicine was outlawed that society became plagued with so many chronic diseases, disorders, and complications.

Look around and you will find that what is bad and outright dangerous is made to appear good and beneficial, and what is good and wholesome is vehemently attacked, discredited, and outlawed. Take for example the idea that synthetic Vitamin C is more beneficial than a fresh orange. Marketing propaganda has many convinced that the over the counter Vitamin C pill which is made of synthetic petroleum based chemical compounds are every bit as good for you or even better. We only need to listen to our intuition to know that this is completely absurd! Unfortunately, many accept this and other similar deceptions on a daily basis when it comes to what they choose to consume as well as what they put on their largest eliminative organ, their skin.

Did you know that most synthetic medicines are derived from petroleum products? This little known fact explains why it is a **multi-billion** dollar industry. Pfizer[1] is actually the largest of the pharmaceutical/petrochemical companies, currently valued at around 265 billion dollars. So not only do these same companies own the pharmacies and the drug stores, but they also contribute billions of dollars into the education[2] (or miseducation) of medical doctors. Through the AMA (American Medical Association) doctors are taught that these toxic drugs are better, safer and more

---

[1] The Investment 'Business With Disease' by Chris Fairhurst, The Hague Tribunal, June 13, 2003
[2] Non-Profit Organizations With Ties to Industry, Integrity in Science, A CSPI Project (www.cspinet.org)

economical than natural remedies. You see, since nothing in nature can be patented, they have been unable to corner the natural herbs market and make billions. Their only recourse is to discredit ALL natural healing modalities as being ineffective and dangerous. They have even gone as far as targeting anyone who openly claims that anything found in nature has the ability to heal and cure dis-ease.

In sharp contrast, the synthetic toxic drugs created in their labs are patented and sold with limited safety trials, despite their harmful side effects. By making the masses believe that anything natural is ineffective and harmful, they have succeeded in getting millions to willingly give up their autonomy and run to their medical professionals for a drug prescription at the first sign of any discomfort or illness.

As a society in general, we are often stuck in a rut as it were. Most of us are eating non-foods, while consuming dangerous and toxic drugs that only serve as a band-aid to our growing health issues. The truth is that one cannot truly have a good life without first achieving good health. For that reason, it is imperative that we focus on taking care of our bodies holistically, by eating nourishing foods, paying attention to what we feed our minds, and getting adequate exercise.

Yes, it is time we go back to basics if we want to attain better physical, emotional, and spiritual health. Let us not ignore the abundant resources provided in nature for healing the mind, body, and spirit. Our efforts for doing so will pay some of the biggest dividends that we will ever enjoy.

I want to share with you my own personal journey, in the hopes that it motivates you to consider the lasting benefits that come with relying on holistic measures for nourishing and healing our bodies. This book will provide you with usable knowledge in regards to the preparation and use of common herbs, as well as give you ideas and practical suggestions on how you can take crucial steps towards a healthier life by making mindful adjustments to how you nourish your body through the food you consume and what you put on your skin.

Chapter 2
My Story

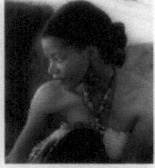

Many would agree that at the rate we are going, in order to save ourselves from extinction, we must be willing to make radical changes now in how we view the human body and its way of healing. Thomas Edison wisely once said that 'the doctor of the future will give no medicine but will interest his patients in the care of the human frame, in diet and in the cause and prevention of disease'. I am hopeful that the type of medicine that will survive into the future will be that which is natural and non-aggressive in nature.

Can you imagine our children or grandchildren living in a time when they will not have to be cut or drugged in order to be healed? I know this idea might sound radical and utopian to some. And please don't misunderstand me here. I will be the first to say that surgery certainly does have its place in medicine, but definitely NOT in the curative or preventative context. Just look around you and consider how many young women are being talked into having their breasts and reproductive parts removed, when they do not even have cancer yet, simply because they believe a certain illness runs in the family.

There is no doubt that there is a great need for us to connect with nature again, if we are to be set free from the misleading advertising and negative programming that has dulled our senses and pushed us to let go of common sense. We need to acknowledge that the body, mind, and spirit are connected and that the body, or its symptoms of illness, cannot be treated in parts. When we begin to understand that the body functions as a whole unit, we begin to understand that dis-ease cannot simply be cut out. It is important that people know there are alternatives and other ways of pursuing wellness; and for that to take place, re-education is essential!

I want to share with you my own personal story because I believe it would be beneficial for others to know what led me on this path and why I am so passionate about herbs and natural living. I believe that my personal experiences and challenges were the catalyst that put me on the road to wellness and opened me up to live my purpose. My desire is that these personal lessons serve as motivation to others.

Rose Hips vs. Synthetic Vit C

It might surprise you to know that Rose Hips are extremely high in natural Vitamin C. Many other herbs like Parsley are actually full of Vitamin C as well, but Rose Hips in particular contain approximately 1,800 milligrams of Vitamin C (this is the equivalent of 20 oranges!). So which would you prefer? The synthetic chemically enhanced form of Vitamin C or the natural form with no side effects. If our end goal is continued wellness, it should be obvious which one our body would benefit the most from.

Shortly after getting married, my husband and I wanted to start our family so we both agreed that I would stop taking birth control pills. We were relatively young - I was 32 and he was 38 - and we were both in seemingly great health. We expected it to be easy. However, after the third miscarriage I started to have my doubts. In fact, during my fourth miscarriage, my ob-gyn told me she could do nothing further for me and referred me to several fertility specialists in the area.

I wasted no time in contacting them and making the necessary appointments. In short order we began to be bounced around from specialist to specialist (five in total), for almost an entire year. It is mostly a distant memory for me now, however, my notes, which consist of several binders' worth of medical reports and hand written notes indicate that the experts initially suspected a luteal phase defect[3]. A second specialist suspected a MTHFR

---

[3] A luteal phase defect is a disruption in a woman's monthly cycle, where the lining of the uterus does not grow properly each month. This can make it difficult to become or remain pregnant.

mutation[4] as well as a possible blood clotting disorder known as thrombophilia.

Even my husband was subjected to numerous tests, in order to rule out whether or not he was the source of the problem. In addition, after almost a year of undergoing tests, fertility drugs and countless procedures including blood tests to determine the problem, it was beyond frustrating, when every single test came back normal. After nearly a year, not one of those experts was able to tell us conclusively what our problem was.

Now I am not undermining those experts and their usefulness in certain cases. In fact, I do realize that there are some couples for whom the process is completely different and they are able to pin point some type of issue and go on to have children whether naturally or by artificial means. But, I have to balance that acknowledgement with the reality that there are many more couples like my husband and I, that go through a great deal, and do not get any answers in the end; couples whose optimism and joy at the prospect of becoming parents were overshadowed by the idea that there was something wrong with their reproductive abilities; couples whose marriage started to become strained because not having the answers they hoped to get from the experts ultimately took a toll on their marriage in terms of how they related to each other and their respective ability to deal with the disappointment and heartache involved. In retrospect, it is also quite telling how not one of those experts ever felt it relevant or necessary to ask any questions about 'us', about our daily habits, our lifestyle, our diet, etc. It seems that the human being (i.e., the individual) is not at all relevant in their standard model of care.

As you would imagine, we were both emotionally and physically drained from the bi-weekly appointments, the lack of answers, and all of the uncertainty. We both decided that a break was needed. We needed a break from doctors, from fertility tests, the constant blood work, the fertility drugs and from family planning. We shifted our focus to personal and household projects

---

[4]MTHFR is a genetic variant which impairs the ability for the body to process folate (B Vitamins). This often leads to elevated levels of homocysteine in some people. High homocysteine levels are common in individuals with kidney disease, low levels of thyroid hormones, psoriasis.

that we had been neglecting for months. It was during this break that I got pregnant again. Funny how that works, right? This would be my fifth pregnancy. What I did not know at the time was that the fertility drugs that they had given me two months prior to monitor my luteal phase were still very much in my system. Imagine our shock when we were told during the first routine ultra sound that we were pregnant with triplets! As you will soon see, this fifth pregnancy proved to be the most challenging experience I have had to date, in my quest for motherhood.

During our second office visit, we were told that only two heartbeats were detected. As awful as it may sound, this was somewhat of a relief. Having twins was still a daunting prospect, but not nearly as frightening as having triplets. Our specialists felt we had progressed enough under their care to ensure a live birth, and so after the eighth week the specialists released us to our new high risk ob-gyn, who also happened to be a distant relative. Under the care of our new high-risk doctor, the pregnancy seemed to progress well. After the fourth month, we finally allowed ourselves to get excited and began to share the news with our immediate family and close friends.

At about 17 weeks gestation I had a routine appointment with my doctor. I recall that he did a pelvic exam. To this day, I do not understand the 'why' of that exam. He took a blood and urine sample and confirmed everything was going along beautifully. There were no concerns whatsoever on his part. What happened the next day is vividly engraved in my mind. It was a beautiful sunny Thursday; I even remember what I was wearing. Since it was such a beautiful day, I decided to take a short walk during my lunch break. After leaving the office for the day, I decided to stop by the local market to pick up a few things. As I was exiting my vehicle, I noticed what seemed like mild pelvic pressure. I was feeling great otherwise, so I quickly dismissed it. When I reached home the pelvic pressure had increased significantly. So much so that I decided to sit and put my feet up for a minute. It was at this point that I felt and heard a pop; my mucous plug was released and a great deal of fluid started gushing out. I was home alone and naturally started to panic. I grabbed the phone and ran to the bathroom to call my husband who was nearly an hour away. Knowing that he would not reach home in time, he contacted a friend at the local police department who immediately dispatched an ambulance on my behalf. I remained on the phone with him until the ambulance arrived.

Once at the hospital, I was observed for a few days and since there was no significant change for the worse, I was released and told by my doctor to fully expect my body to go into what they call 'automatic abortion mode'. I will admit that although I heard and understood the words, I truly had no idea what that process would be like. What I do know is that within 48 hours my body was in full labor. I called my doctor for guidance and he suggested that I ride it out and drink a glass of wine. Seriously! I endured the pains (without the wine) and after almost four hours of non-stop contractions, I was finally able to catch my breath. At about three in the morning, I got up to urinate in a bedpan that my husband loving placed on the side of the bed so that I would not have to walk the distance to the bathroom. I remember feeling a very unusual sensation as my muscles started to contract to release the urine flow. I suddenly felt something heavy slide out of me and at that instant I knew what it was. It was so surreal and yet I was surprisingly calm. At this point my lifeless baby (Baby A) was hanging outside of my body by the umbilical cord. I called out to my husband who was asleep. He frantically managed to put a skirt on me and helped me get in the car (with the baby held in a plastic bag between my legs). It all felt like a very bad nightmare that we just could not wake from.

> Chickweed is a useful source of Vitamin C, and it is delicious, when consumed in salads or cooked as a vegetable.

My doctor was not available when we arrived at the hospital, so I was attended to by a very young emergency room intern who nonchalantly proceeded to cut the umbilical cord and placed the body of my lifeless baby in a bright red specimen bag labeled 'hazardous'. It all felt like it was happening in slow motion. Finally, when my doctor arrived, several hours later, he urged us to consider terminating our remaining baby (Baby B) immediately. After discussing it in private, we decided to go against his recommendation to terminate. We opted to allow nature to run its course. As you would imagine, we received a tremendous amount of resistance from the medical professionals for making this decision.

My husband and I were determined to let things be primarily because it was his professional opinion my life or immediate health were not in any danger.

In case you are wondering, we did not have false hopes that our second baby would make it through such a stressful ordeal. We were prepared for the worst but strongly believed that allowing things to end naturally would at the very least honor both of our sons. We felt that was the least we could do given the difficult circumstances. In the end, our second son survived until just 25 weeks. I experienced a significant amount of bleeding during which time his little heart gave out under the stress. I recall how the doctor asked me whether I wanted to be placed under general anesthesia in order to have the baby removed from my body via c-section, as opposed to having labor induced with Pitocin. There is no doubt in my mind that in suggesting the c-section, he was trying to be sensitive to my emotional well-being. I will admit that it was a tempting proposition, but one I quickly rejected. I knew that despite the emotional pain involved, I wanted to have all of my senses during this bitter sweet experience. Even though I would not be able to deliver a live baby, I wanted to remember he was once very much alive and growing inside me. I wanted to honor his brief existence by allowing him to pass through my birth canal the way he would have, if he were alive. It was a very challenging day for the both of us. While I remained in the hospital recuperating, he arranged to have my placenta and the baby's body retrieved from the hospital by a local funeral home. We opted to have both cremated and a portion of the baby's ashes where spread near the roots of a cherry blossom tree that we planted in our backyard. To this day, that blossom tree is the strongest and most beautiful tree in that yard.

I was in the hospital on strict bed rest for approximately two months during this entire experience. It was during that hospital stay that I began to see how little say the patient has on the course of treatment given, and how much resistance is unleashed when what the patient demands does not benefit the hospital financially. I also witnessed how most of the decisions made by the medical staff are more often than not, based on 'liability and risk', because at the end of the day, it is a business.

Through my involvement in several loss support groups and based on my own experience, it became clear to me that the emotional toll of such a loss is always far greater than the physical. Long after I recovered physically, my heart still ached and some days were harder than others. I especially remember how difficult it was for me when I approached my due date. It was as if an overwhelming flood of raw emotions consumed every fiber of my body on a daily basis. The emotional pain was almost paralyzing. I am not sure exactly when I stood up, picked my heart up from the floor and said "enough", but thankfully, I did reach that point. I began to quickly transform my grief into an unbridled determination and focus to find real answers. I intuitively started to research more and more about nutrition, Ayurvedic medicine, homeopathy, herbs, traditional foods, and natural remedies. I was a human sponge willing to consider and absorb anything and everything outside of the mainstream box. I joined an online support group that introduced me to the Weston A. Price Foundation and its amazing nutritional principles. I researched naturopaths in our area and wasted no time in making an appointment to see one. Upon meeting with the naturopath, I was astonished to find that after only two visits and only one round of blood work -compared to the several gallons of blood I had given to

Effective combinations:

For lymphatic health, Cleavers will work well with Echinacea. For skin issues, it is best combined with Burdock.

the previous team of allopathic specialists - the naturopath was able to tell me more than an entire room of medical experts could in a year. Based on the results of my blood work he was able to tell me in detail exactly what my body was lacking and the foods and supplements I needed to introduce into my system, in order to heal. Briefly, the naturopath's assessment was that my adrenals and thyroid glands were not functioning properly. He thus suggested that they become my primary focus in my quest for healing.

While researching, I learned that more than 75% of women are considered estrogen dominant and discovered that females produce estrogen primarily in four places; the liver, fat cells, ovaries and adrenal glands. It is this abnormal spike in estrogen that often causes ovarian cysts, premature births, infertility, fibroids, painful and excessive bleeding during our menstrual cycle, hair loss, low libido, etc. High estrogen levels result in low progesterone, which in turn drains the adrenals and thyroid. When our adrenals and thyroid are not functioning properly, the hormones needed to create and support a new life are also out of balance and that is when this imbalance manifests itself in the form of infertility. This hormonal imbalance is caused by different factors, but the biggest culprits typically are:

> Birth control pills;
> Hormones present in commercial meats, dairy products,
> Processed non-foods;
> Pesticides in vegetation;
> Bath and beauty products;
> Toxins in our environment.

The list of changes I wanted to implement based on this newly found information was daunting, but I was ready to begin. My first task was clearing out our pantry and removing all processed and packaged foods, white sugar, white flour and snacks from our home. I simply started from scratch, leaving only the raw basics. I immediately started following a nutritional plan specifically designed for pre-conception that is encouraged by the West A. Price Foundation. I increased my green foods intake, started taking coconut oil, raw (pastured) egg yolks, as well as other super foods and herbal tinctures daily. There are other changes that I made which I will get into in detail in a later chapter, but after about two months on this new regimen, I started to witness a change in my physical health. I had more energy, more mental clarity, my sleep pattern improved; my bowel movements became regular, my skin cleared up, and my mood and overall attitude shifted for the better.

As I experienced these positive changes, I slowly began to grasp the connection between my current health and my prior food choices, my thinking, my extended use of birth control years prior, and even my spirituality. I finally started to understand that the body, mind, and spirit connection cannot be ignored if one seeks holistic wellness – each part must be addressed in order for us to truly heal. At this point, it was as if a light bulb went off in my head and everything started to make sense. I began to see how little most medically trained doctors know about wellness and prevention and was surprised to learn what the actual amount of contact hours a typical medical doctor receives in nutrition during their four years or more in medical school. The national average came out to be about 10 hours![5] Therefore, unless they decide to specialize in nutrition (and we can safely say that is rare because it is not where the money is), the average doctor has less than half a day's worth of time spent learning about how to keep your body functioning properly with the right foods. I routinely spend more than that reading nutrition, herbs and wellness related articles and books in a one-week period. How are you possibly supposed to learn everything you need to know about proper nutrition in 10 hours? The answer is you can't. Not only that, but how much of those 10 hours of nutritional training will they remember? Not many in all likelihood, unless they continually review them. With very few exceptions, the average physician (from surgeon to general practitioner) specializes in nothing more than illness, disease, injuries, and medication.

After about six months on this strict pre-conception regimen, I became pregnant with my first living child. This pregnancy was challenging in many ways because I was still under the care of the same high-risk doctor. My mind had shifted significantly, as I increased in knowledge, but I was still largely controlled by fear; fear of another loss. I was not yet grounded enough in my conviction to know with every fiber of my being, that I would have a different outcome this time around. So as a result, I allowed a lot of unnecessary intervention (i.e., ultra sounds, tests and useless medical drugs) during that pregnancy. I was put on bed rest when I entered my third trimester, not because of any complication, but rather as a precaution simply due to my 'high risk' status. My beautiful daughter Mikaelah arrived at 36 weeks via c-section. Moreover, although it was not the type of birthing experience I had envisioned, we were beyond thrilled to finally be able to hold our baby in our arms.

---

[5] Status of Nutrition Education in Medical Schools, by Kelly M. Adams, et al, The American Journal of Clinical Nutrition, Am J Clin Nutr, April 2006, Vol. 82, no. 49415-9445

If you fast-forward two years to my next pregnancy with my son, and you were to ask me what that pregnancy was like, I would describe it as blissful from beginning to end. It truly was! By this time, I had completely stepped into my power as a woman and was quite confident in my natural choices and in my body's ability to sustain a life. In anticipation of this pregnancy, I read a lot and prepared myself emotionally, mentally and spiritually for the type of pregnancy I knew I could experience and deserved. I enlisted the support of two very experienced midwives who allowed me to enjoy a pregnancy where I felt honored, supported and empowered the entire time. I made a concerted effort to surround myself with nurturing emotional support.

During this pregnancy, I quickly but lovingly corrected anyone that (even if with good intentions) tried to encourage me by somehow interjecting negative talk or even bringing my prior losses into the conversation. This time around I knew that the energy within my body was affected by the energy around me and more importantly, how I related to it all. I also grew into the understanding that if my way of living and thinking was not life-affirming, that the systems in my body dedicated to the creation of a new life would be adversely affected. And so for this reason, I passionately refused to allow anyone to project their negative thoughts onto my pregnancy experience. This time around, there was no fear. I was quite determined to protect my mental and emotional space to ensure a peaceful and blissful welcome for my baby.

My purpose in sharing my story with you is to uplift and encourage you. If you have doubts about whether natural healing will truly benefit you and your family, or if you feel that you do not yet know enough to take control of your health, start now! In addition, be confident in the fact that if the desire is there, you can and you will! If like many you think that only medically trained professionals should have a say in our wellness because after all, they are the ones with the medical training, I am here to tell you that you have been misled. In fact, I would respectfully say that it is this type of thinking that has created an extremely weak, ignorant and very dependent consciousness, when it comes to looking after the health of our own bodies. Because people no longer want to take responsibility for their wellness, they are generally completely out of touch with their bodies and their emotional state.

As I have mentioned earlier, I do believe that medical doctors are useful. Their medical training is particularly useful for surgery and in instances of an emergency where there are broken bones, life-threatening injuries, wounds with excessive bleeding, and so forth. However, the idea that one needs to rely on a medical surgeon (which is what most AMA trained doctors are) to maintain wellness is not one I subscribe to. I would also like to say that I have the utmost respect for medical professionals that look at the patient/doctor relationship as a partnership. There are doctors that recognize that as the patient, it is your body (or that of your child's) and that you (the patient/parent) have the final say on what goes on in any medical situation, even when that choice goes against their professional medical advice. I have had the pleasure of dealing with several medically trained doctors that took a holistic approach when dealing with their patients and they were like a breath of fresh air. However, the sad reality is that while they do exist, open-minded medical professionals that hold to this basic tenet are too far in between. That is precisely why I say that *knowledge is power*. Once you become aware that you do have a choice, that realization coupled with determination is enough to change the world.

Aside from my own experience, I have personally witnessed over the years many people close to me hand over their personal power and their common sense to 'professionals' that really do not know how to cure them of their ills. Repeatedly I have observed how many are unable or unwilling to take personal responsibility for themselves or their health issues. Instead, they become willing research participants for the sick care industry, resulting in the deterioration and decline of their health and overall quality of life. This has been quite painful to witness, especially when you make a great effort to help someone see the benefits that can be experienced from living holistically. However, I balance that disappointment with the understanding that we all come to this information at different stages and it is only meant for us to fully grasp and embrace, when we are receptive to it on a spiritual level.

I will be the first to admit that it is quite an uncomfortable task to have to examine our own destructive habits and actions and come to the realization that we are causing our own demise by going against what is natural, simply because it is more convenient. It is an even more difficult task to find the courage and determination to go against the norm and implement those much needed lifestyle changes.

It is my heartfelt desire that the information shared in this book encourages you and motivates you to take small steps, which will allow you to heal yourself and your family naturally, on a deep and lasting level. Do it for yourself, for your family, for your children, because you are ALL worth it!

Chapter 3
How Diet Affects Your Healing

I have collected quite a few herbal books over the years and the one thing I have consistently noticed is how none of these books elaborate on the importance of maintaining a nutrient dense diet, when one is seeking to use herbal or other natural remedies to heal from dis-ease. Some of them do briefly mention how using herbs and eating healthy go hand in hand, but there is no further emphasis or guidance given to educate the reader in this very important aspect of the healing process.

I strongly believe that if people knew just how much their diet affected their ability to heal themselves (with or without herbs), they would be more willing to consider it as an option before resorting to drastic measures. Therefore, before we start talking about herbs, I want to take a moment to discuss the impact that maintaining a good diet has on your healing and on your overall wellness.

I am not a nutritional expert by any means, but I have learned quite a bit over the years about traditional nutrient dense foods and about non-foods. I have witnessed firsthand the power that real food has in healing the human body. This correlation is so important that I will go as far as to say that in most cases, our day-to-day dietary habits dictate whether any natural therapy we attempt will work on our behalf.. Using herbs for healing while maintaining a SAD (standard American diet) is like pouring precious jewels down the drain. In short order, you

Our Colon

The colon is responsible for the elimination of toxins and waste the body does not use. When our colon gets backed-up (much like a pipe in your home), pockets of decaying matter form and that is when degenerating dis-ease begins. Some forms of cancers, Candida, and other degenerating dis-ease all start in the colon. Chronic constipation can potentially cause very serious problems in malabsorption, which leads to malnutrition. So even though an individual is eating – and possibly eating very well – food is just not being absorbed properly.

It is important to always target the colon when dealing with any illness. There are certain herbs that have laxative properties, which help stimulate bowel movements. Get to know them!

will become frustrated at the lack of results and dismiss these powerful herbs as being ineffective.

Herbs heal, but they are not a magic pill. Herbs do not work as a band aid, masking the symptoms and making the person think that the issue has been resolved. Unlike allopathic drugs, herbs work in a holistic way by influencing every system of the body, thereby getting to the root cause of the disturbance. The more toxic the body, the longer it will take to see positive results when working with herbs. So please remember, our nutrition must be of a quality that enables the body to renew itself in a way that ensures health and wholeness. This means that we must educate ourselves in nutritional habits that promote wellness so that once healed, the body will not succumb to illness again.

The human body is amazing. When we take care of it, it acts as a self-healing machine with a wonderfully effective and even astounding mechanism for eliminating waste and poisons. On the other hand, when we don't value it, a poor diet will bring to the surface symptoms that are somewhat moderate (i.e., headaches, constipation, gas, nervousness, excitability, etc.). These seemingly mild symptoms are the early signals that our body gently gives us when letting us know that something is out of balance. Much like a car's warning light will turn on letting us know what needs to be repaired. If these warning signals are ignored, they can and will develop into very dangerous complications such as diabetes, high blood pressure, heart disease and cancer. For this reason, it is important to emphasize that a well nourished body has the necessary reserves to suppress and destroy malignancies. Conversely, a malnourished body will succumb to disease and the eventual deterioration of vital organs. You are what you eat!

So *where does one start*? Based on everything we have discussed so far, it might seem over-whelming but I encourage you to keep reading. As you go through this book, make a list of what changes you can easily implement now, and be determined to start there.

There are many diets promoted today and sometimes it is confusing to discern which one of them will actually lead to optimal health. There is veganism, raw foodism, vegetarianism, paleoism, and the list goes on. Some individuals are motivated to follow these diets because of certain health concerns, or simply to be able to reach a certain goal, such as releasing weight. I will not get into promoting one diet over another because it truly is a personal choice. I will say this however: be careful not to get caught up with fads or labels. Whatever your diet choice, always make your intention and your desired end result a happier, healthier and more balanced you.

Whatever eating regimen you choose, what should be constant is your focus to eat as much fresh fruits and vegetables as your budget will allow, and as little processed and packaged foods as possible. My personal mantra is "cook your food". You may find as I did, that if you make an effort to eat as little processed and packaged foods as possible, the upside will be that you will be forced to think about what you are putting on your family's dinner table. Furthermore, when we start to look at food more consciously and as a means to maintain health, we will instinctively start to "eat to live" and not "live to eat".

When I started on the journey to heal my body after my losses, I briefly adopted a vegetarian lifestyle. I benefited a great deal from that dietary change, as my body seriously needed to detox and get back into balance (physically and mentally). However, after I accomplished my goal, I decided to incorporate some grass fed animal protein back into my diet. You see, raw and vegetarian diets are most effective for my body-type when what I desire is a short-term detox or cleanse. My husband and I both try to do short-term juice cleanses at least once a year in order to give our bodies a fresh start. Again, whatever diet you choose, make sure that it works for your body on a holistic level.

Microwaves and Food

A clinical research study was done by a Swiss scientist, *Dr. Hans Hertel,* on the effects of microwave-processed food on the human body. That study determined that microwaves violently vibrate the water molecules in food, thus creating internal friction and heating the food from the inside out, while other forms of heat, including the sun do not create friction heat in organic substances. The radiation, created by microwaves, results in the destruction and deformation of food molecules, plus the formation of new compounds, which are substances that are formed through the subjection to radiation. Is it possible, that we are ignorantly sacrificing health on the altar of convenience?

● ● ●

24

Pay attention to how you feel, your thoughts, your emotions, and how your body functions while on the diet. Ask yourself, do I feel lethargic? Do I have more energy? Do I feel good? Allow your body to give you the feedback you need in order to determine if that particular dietary regimen is working for you. If it is not working for you, make the adjustments necessary and move onto one that does.

Our bodies are indeed complex; however, what it needs from us in order to function properly is often quite simple:

1.   Wholesome Nutrition.   Whenever possible, choose real foods over processed dead foods. Eat as much green vegetables and fresh fruits as possible. Avoid packaged and processed foods. Avoid coffee, alcohol, drugs, soft-drinks, artificial preservatives and synthetic sweeteners (i.e., Truvia, Sweet & Low, and High Fructose Corn Syrup). And more importantly, get into the habit of reading labels! In addition, as a side note: If you are raising a family, when your children see you reading labels, they will start to do it too. My children will not eat anything outside the home until they can verify with me that the ingredients are wholesome. One of the immediate benefits I see with this practice is that from a very young age they become aware of how food affects their bodies. This is a good habit that will serve them well long after they leave your nest. Remember that if your body is fed toxic food and indigestible things such as sugary sweets and processed foods, it will be unable to fight infection when necessary. Treat your body well by regularly giving it nourishing foods, and it will take care of you and support you when you need it to.

2.   Rest. Proper rest and good health go hand in hand. Yet, if you are anything like me, good solid rest is likely the one thing you never get enough of. When we get our needed rest we allow our body to regenerate itself on a cellular level. Our body does not function properly if it is in a constant state of tension. In a later chapter, I will share with you an herbal bath infusion that may be used to relax the body and mind after a long day and is an excellent way to promote restful sleep. Depriving our body from the time it needs to heal is detrimental to our health. If getting a good night sleep is an issue for you, you will likely benefit from the non-habit forming herbal tincture found in the 'Herbal Remedies' section. This simple

and effective tincture will aid you or your loved ones with insomnia and will promote restful sleep.

3.   Cleansing. Periodic cleanses give the body's systems a boost and the colon benefits immensely from a cleanse. If you suffer from chronic constipation (which I did for years), it would be worth researching how a temporary juice fast (with gentle fruits and vegetables) might benefit you. Herbs and a good diet are helpful, but unless the body is actually able to eliminate accumulated toxic waste via regular bowel movements, then all of your efforts will be in vain. This toxic waste will continue to be reabsorbed into your body's systems, making your chronic condition worse. There are certain detoxifying herbs that have a good effect on digestion and on the intestines, which will aid you in becoming regular. I encourage you to become familiar with the herbs listed in the Herbal Index section, on *Page 45*.

4.   Exercise. Exercise does not have to be uncomfortable or painful. I have never been extremely athletic, but having two small children and living on a farm affords me more than enough opportunities to be active. In fact, some days I go to bed sore from the mere task of tending to our animals and keeping up with the children. I especially enjoy nature walks, yoga, and a good lymphatic workout with my children in the trampoline. You do not need to run five miles a day or even be inside a gym facility daily to accomplish this. Just find an activity that you enjoy and that works with your lifestyle. As with anything, moderation and consistency is important. Always remember that you should feel energized and charged after a workout, not exhausted and in pain.

಄಄

Our Thoughts Matter!

Are your thoughts making you sick? Did you know that a major cause of illness is the misuse of the mind? Negative thought forms and mental upsets can cause disease. Sorrowful, hateful, and negative outlooks cause toxic chemicals to be released inside the physical body. This in turn creates an imbalance and a constant state of toxic chemical secretions, causing the person to manifest some type of illness. The illness will vary, but the cause is always the same. Learn to control your mind and you may very well have found the key to wellness!

಄಄

It is also important for me to mention that our biggest ally in healing is our mind. It has been observed that a person's general outlook and disposition in regards to life in general often will affect their health and how quickly their body heals when they are faced with an illness. I have experienced this first hand, as well as witnessed it in others.

We have often heard it said that we are what we eat. But we are also what we breathe, what we think, what we say and what we see. We have already touched on the importance of wholesome food and exercise. Naturally, it is quite easy for us to associate those two things with our health because they do go hand in hand. However, what about the books that we choose to read? the films and television we watch? the politics we support? Is the music we listen to good for our health? Are our friends good for us? These are very personal but very relevant questions which will undoubtedly elicit different answers from each one of us. Whatever the response, do not ignore it; be very aware that those things also have a bearing on your wellbeing.

The most fascinating and meaningful realization for me in this journey has been the fact that in holistic health each individual has the capacity for self-healing. The person who is ill is in fact the healer. There is so much power in those words because while assistance may be provided from outside sources (i.e., medical experts, supportive friends and family, etc.), the responsibility for healing lies with the person who wants to be well. Your thoughts and actions are what will make it manifest. There is no denying that using herbs and wholesome nutrition to that end is an ideal way to co-operate with your own innate healing power. This type of knowledge is empowering!

Chapter 4
How I Got Started

I understand firsthand how modifying our lifestyle might seem overwhelming at first. It is often difficult to know where to start. I want to share with you the changes that my family and I made over the course of time. Please remember that these are in no way intended as dietary recommendations. I encourage you to do what you are called to do in this regard. More importantly, I urge you to research everything that is mentioned in this book, before you decide to adopt it as part of your family's routine. I will share what has worked for my family and hope that you find the information beneficial in your journey:

1.   Beverages - Before having our children, we were big on soft-drinks. Our pantry was never short of what is often referred to as 'liquid crack'. After learning that some studies suggest a link between drinking soda and obesity, tooth decay, weaker bones and even brain development in children[6], I began substituting coffee, tea, processed fruit juices, soft-drinks and other sugary drinks with home brewed herbal teas, home brewed kombucha (a probiotic drink), home brewed kefir water and water. Now we consume home brewed kombucha, kefir water, lemon infused water and herbal infusions on a daily basis. We avoid tap water as it is often chemically treated with chlorine and fluoride, which are both damaging to the body. Many studies have shown that fluoride accumulates and calcifies the pineal gland. The pineal gland in the brain releases the hormone melatonin, which controls our sleep patterns. In the first published fluoridation safety experiment in Newburgh, New York, the authors found that girls living in a fluoridated community reached puberty five months earlier than girls living in a non-fluoridated community. My research proved to be compelling enough to motivate me to purchase a portable Berkey water filter with a fluoride attachment to remove fluoride and most other harmful substances. I will provide the information of where we purchased our portable water filer in the Resources section

---

[6] The Effects of Caffeine on Sleep and Maturational Markers in Rat, by Nadja Olini, Salome Kurth and Reto Huber, www.plosone.org, September 4, 2013, DOI:10.1371/journal.pone.0072539

(Page 120). If you are unsure as to whether your local municipality adds fluoride to your water supply, you should contact them directly to confirm it. This is public information that would be readily available to you upon inquiry.

2.   Dairy products - I gave up processed milk, cheese, and yogurt and started consuming raw milk, raw cheese, and raw yogurt. Unless you have been living under a rock, I am sure you are aware or at least have heard of the huge controversy surrounding raw milk. It is my opinion that raw milk that comes from pastured, healthy, hormone-free cows is unparalleled to pasteurized hormone and antibiotic laden commercial milk. I have been consuming raw milk for over seven years and would rather forgo milk altogether than go back to commercially processed milk (including any of its processed by-products). The dangers posed by commercial milk, as it pertains to our growing children and their premature development are very real. I encourage you to research the subject so that you are better able to make an informed decision, if this does in fact apply to you and your family. The Weston A. Price Foundation is a good place to start, as this organization has been doing amazing work in their efforts to educate families on the benefits of raw dairy and traditional nutrient dense foods for healing. I will include their

Effective combinations:

As a natural antibiotic Echinacea may be combined with Goldenseal. When combined with Yarrow it will effectively stop cystitis.

information in the Resources section of this book (Page 120).

3.   Breads - This was easy to give up once I learned that commercial breads (and even those sold at supermarket bakeries) are loaded with preservatives and artificial additives like potassium bromine[7], which inhibits metabolism, and is a known cancer causing agent, which is also found in pesticides. This toxic ingredient is used in bread for the mere task of ensuring a perfect loaf in every batch. I have since learned how to make our own bread using organic, unbleached and un-bromated flour. In the rare occasion that I have

---

[7] Elevated bromide [bromine] levels have been implicated in every thyroid disease, from simple hypothyroidism to autoimmune diseases to thyroid cancer. – Bromide Dominance Theory – How Competitive Inhibition Causes Deficiency, by Lynne Farow 2007

to go outside to source bread, I make it a point to source bread that is made without bromated flour. You might also be surprised to know that bromine is found in anti-depressants, mattresses, sodas, Gatorade, cosmetics, prescription drugs, asthma inhalers, and fabric softeners.

4.   Cereals – Although many of us grew up eating them, the truth is that most, if not all packaged cereals lack nutritional substance. All packaged cereals are produced by a process called "extrusion".   Extrusion involves high heat and high pressure in order to form the grain into those pretty and popular shapes like the Os and flakes. This process also destroys most of the nutrients, including the synthetic chemical vitamins that are often added to "fortify" the cereal. Extrusion especially ravages amino acids (the building blocks of protein), rendering them highly toxic. During this process, protein structures are altered, and as a result, foreign compounds form, which are potentially harmful and definitely not part of a balanced breakfast. What about the high fiber, 'organic' cereals made from 'healthier' grains? These are often marketed as the best nutritional choice because these cereals tend to have more protein than conventional dry packaged cereals. However, when the high-protein grains are extruded, they produce even more denatured protein and are very difficult for the body to digest. Therefore, your "healthy" cereal is potentially worse for you than junk cereals, since they contain more high-protein grains that have been ultra-processed. For those compelling reasons, I now make my own granola or use only whole and ancient grains like steel cut oatmeal, millet, quinoa, etc.

5.   Eggs – It is no secret that much like the meat available in supermarkets today, commercial eggs are also full of additives, hormones, and antibiotics. We now keep chickens for eggs. However, before we had our hens, we sourced local free range, antibiotic free eggs from neighboring farmers. It may seem like quite the effort to find free range eggs especially when you live in suburbia, but I was really surprised at how many local resources I had available to me in my area when I did a quick online search. Check the Resources section of this book found on *Page 120*, for links on where to go to start your own search.

6.   Fruits and Vegetables - I do my best to eat whatever is in season and available locally. I no longer purchase canned fruits or vegetables. On occasion, I will purchase frozen organic fruits and vegetables if it is on sale. When my family's budget does not allow for organic produce, I do buy conventional. However, I place all fruits and vegetables in a large water-filled bowl (enough to cover veggies or fruit) and add about 2 tablespoons of raw apple cider vinegar. I allow them to soak for about 15 minutes and then rinse before consuming. The apple cider vinegar helps to break down or dissolve toxic wax and pesticides.

7.   Legumes - I no longer purchase canned beans. I buy everything dried and make sure I soak them overnight before cooking, in order to aid the digestion and absorption process after consuming.

8.   Rice – Rice is a regular staple in our household. I prefer to use brown rice, basmati or jasmine and buy organic if my budget allows. I avoid bleached, enriched, starched, parboiled, instant, or pre-seasoned rice, which are full of harmful preservatives and chemicals and have little nutritional value.

9.   Pasta - I avoid white flour pasta unless it is organic. If that is not possible due to my budget, I opt for whole grain, rice pasta, brown rice pasta, or spelt pasta, which is much easier for the body to digest.

10.   Meat, Fish & Poultry - We consume meat about twice a week. I source our meat locally from neighbors that are ethical farmers. We are fortunate to live in a rural area where we have access to several conscientious farmers. However, if we did not have that as an option, we would probably not eat meat at all. I know this sounds drastic, but when one considers how most market meat is injected with growth hormones, toxins, chemicals, antibiotics, and wormers, it is enough for me to want to avoid it. If supermarket meats are the only option available to you, try to select antibiotic and hormone free cuts, which are sometimes available. I personally avoid cured meats and by-products such as hot dogs, cold cuts, corned beef, etc. These contain sodium nitrates and nitrites, which are harmful, and they have been known to contribute to cancer. It is worth remembering that moderation in the consumption of animal protein is always important when one considers the fact that it takes an adult approximately six hours to digest meats and that partially digested proteins are toxic to the body.

Effective Combinations: For skin issues, combine Burdock with Yellow Dock, Red Clover, or Cleavers.

As for fish, my rule of thumb is that the fish or seafood be wild-caught. Farm raised fish is typically enhanced with toxic substances. If I cannot find wild caught fish at a reasonable price, I do without it.

11.   Soups - I avoid soup mixes and canned soups that contain MSG and other harmful preservatives and opt to make my soups at home. I love making bone broths using locally sourced beef bones and chicken bones/feet. Bone broths are super foods in their own right, full of minerals and nutrients that truly heal and help a weak and sickly body. They are incredibly easy to make and they freeze amazingly well and serve as a great base for other dishes.

12.   Sweets/Desserts – My husband and children regularly crave sweets, which is a bit challenging for me, considering I usually prefer fresh fruits to calm any sweet cravings. In order to keep them happy, I make our own cakes, cookies, sweet breads, raw desserts, custards, and ice cream using wholesome and natural ingredients. I will admit that I do have a weakness for premium chocolate and I always stock up whenever I come across a sale. Just remember, you do not have to give up everything that gives you pleasure. Try to find a healthier version of whatever that one thing is that you truly enjoy.

Food and Children

Often times, hyperactive learning disorders in children are caused by allergy or artificial coloring and flavoring agents that are found in processed foods. Things that you may not expect, like commercial ice-cream, cakes, pancakes, margarine, jello, candy, Kool-Aid, fruit juices - they ALL contain artificial additives and chemicals that affect the growing brains of our children. I encourage you to get into the habit of reading labels like your (and your family's) life depended on it... because it does!

13.   Salt/Condiments – Contrary to popular belief, table salt is not just sodium chloride. It also contains additives like aluminum that are designed to make it more free flowing. Ferro cyanide, talc and silica aluminate are commonly included. Aluminum intake leads to neurological disorders, particularly when no selenium is provided to help the body chelate it. Aluminum bio-accumulates inside the body, causing further degeneration over time. Talc is also a known carcinogen so it is worth questioning why the F.D.A. has a special provision to allow talc in table salt, even though it is prohibited in all other foods, due to toxicity issues.   According to current regulations, table salt can be up to 2% talc. Given all of this information, it is certainly wise for anyone seeking good health to avoid it. Without hesitating, I ditched the iodized table salt and now only use real sea salt. I choose real herbs instead of powdered seasonings because of the preservatives and additives they often contain.

14.   Microwave - After doing much research on the effects that microwaving our food has on our health, we decided to dispose of our microwave. There have been controlled studies[8], which have

---

[8] The Proven Dangers of Microwaves, Nexus Magazine, Volume 2, #25 (April-May '95)

shown that microwave cooking changes the molecular structure of your food, as well as your blood to the point that it causes deterioration and an excess of free radicals in the body. Initially, it was difficult not having the convenience of warming up certain foods with the touch of a button, but we quickly realized that not having a microwave gave us an additional incentive to 'cook our food' and eat more consciously.

15.   Personal Care Products - I will admit that making changes in this area was a slow process for me. You see, like many women, I was very much into commercial beauty products. But slowly I started to understand how the multitude of chemicals and hormone disruptors found in many of the beauty products I was accustomed to using, including make-up, contributed towards my endocrine system's imbalance and overall health.

It is my opinion that our collective ignorance as women in this area has damaging consequences and so it is extremely important that I take a brief moment to talk about female personal hygiene products. It was quite disturbing for me to find out through research just how harmful maxi-pads and tampons are to our female reproductive health. For example, did you know that in order to make tampons and maxi pads white, manufacturers add a chemical called Dioxin, which serves to bleach the product? The chemical Dioxin has been linked to endometriosis, pelvic inflammatory disease, breast cancer, estrogen dominant conditions, birth defects in babies, immune system damage, sarcoma, Hodgkin's lymphoma, hormone dysfunction, miscarriage, impaired fertility, lowered concentration ability, diabetes, and impaired thyroid function.

Although levels of Dioxin in tampons and pads are small, and the manufacturers will readily point this out as if to suggest they are safe, they are still quite dangerous, as Dioxin accumulates in the fat stores of the body and can add up to dangerous levels over time. The average woman may have as many as 400 or more periods in her lifetime, and can use up to 15,000 tampons throughout this time. The reality is that out of convenience, most women will opt to use either sanitary pads or tampons, or a combination of both. When you look at it in those terms, you quickly start to see that this is a very large number and that the health implications caused by the toxic products that we as women are choosing to place in our sacred wombs cannot be ignored.

Thankfully, there are more natural and safer alternatives. Washable pads for instance, are made from cotton, hemp, linen, jersey, or wool. They are reusable (which makes them more cost effective) and as an added benefit, they do not pollute the environment. There are also environmentally friendly tampons made of organic cotton, hemp or other fiber, that is grown without the use of herbicides or pesticides and are free of Dioxin, Furans and chlorine bleach.

For the last five years, I have been using a menstrual cup, similar to the well-known Diva cup. Menstrual cups are worn internally like a tampon and are designed to collect the fluid rather than absorb it. They are reusable and typically hold approximately 30 ml of fluid, which is about 1/3 of the average fluid produced in every moon cycle. I remove and empty the cup every three hours (6 to 12 hours is what is recommended) on heavier days. If you are wondering just how effective they are, I have used them on heavier days along with a cloth pad liner and this combination has always provided the extra protection that I needed, even when I was working in a professional environment as a Paralegal. The moon cups are available in latex or medical grade silicone, for those with latex allergies. There are actually two versions available; one for women that have given birth and another for those that have never birthed a child. The cup is easily cleaned with mild soap and water. I allow my moon cup to sit in a water and tea-tree oil solution for a few hours after each cycle. The tea tree oil provides anti-bacterial, anti-fungal, and anti-viral properties that help to disinfect it.

Women must recognize that many of the reproductive challenges we encounter when we finally decide to start our family (i.e., infertility, hormonal imbalance, miscarriages, fibroids, cysts, irregular periods, painful periods, etc.), are simply manifestations of years of continued toxic overload and assault on not only our bodies but also our wombs. This is something that as women we cannot continue to ignore. I challenge every woman not only to educate herself and make better choices in this regard, but also to include her younger daughters, sisters, cousins, nieces, granddaughters, and girlfriends in this important conversation. It is imperative that we educate the younger generation of women coming up. In my case, as is the case with many of the women I have spoken to, my mother or grandmother did not hand down these tools to me. Although a great deal of wisdom could have been imparted in this regard, it seems as if these important topics were almost taboo for most of our mothers and grandmothers. I acknowledge and welcome my responsibility to make sure that my daughter, my son (for he too will one day have a wife), and any receptive young woman that crosses my path, are well aware of these dangers and more importantly, the natural options that they have available to them. It is important that they know that their sacred womb is the source of all life, and as such it should be protected. Once we acknowledge the practical value that this information holds, let us apply it and pass it on as part of a life skills set they will benefit from for years to come.

There is no question that no matter who we are, or where we might live, we are all being bombarded with toxins that are released in the environment on a regular basis. We are often limited as to what we can do to change that, especially when we consider how our own government and big corporations play a major role in this environmental "assault". However, always remember that we are not completely powerless. You do have a say when it comes to personal care products and how you choose to spend your money. Therefore, whether it is deodorant, toothpaste, shower gel, soap or perfume, remember that your power lies in how you choose to spend your dollars. We have often heard it said that when you know better, you do better. Knowledge is power and there is much power in your choice!

I know you are likely thinking that it is impossible to avoid using commercial personal care items. You might also be thinking that the more natural alternatives are just too expensive and therefore out of your reach. However, there is one important thing to remember: you do not have to implement all of these changes at once. It is perfectly fine for you to tackle one personal care item at a time. I found that by learning how to make my own deodorant, toothpaste, lip balms, body lotions, my own moon cycle cloth pads, etc., I was not only being self-sufficient, but I was keeping myself and my family healthy and saving money at the same time. In fact, the desire to help others stay healthy is what motivated me to start my bath and beauty venture, MMSoaps. MMSoaps focuses on providing products that heal the body and skin naturally on a holistic level. I am especially proud of the fact that we have taken the non-conventional route and held true to our mission by refusing to use any synthetic fragrances, lab colors or toxic chemicals when formulating any of our products, no matter how popular these may be with the masses. We value your health as much as we do our own!

As you read this, do not feel overwhelmed and think that you cannot possibly implement everything being shared in this book. My purpose is to raise awareness so that others feel motivated to explore more holistic and healthier options, one step at a time. I encourage you to make a list of what seems reasonable for your lifestyle and be committed to start there. You might find that some of the adjustments I made may not resonate with you and your lifestyle, as they may be too drastic from what you are now used to. Each individual must decide what is best for their bodies and their family and do the best that they can.

> Basil actively inhibits the same enzyme that anti-inflammatory drugs do, including Ibuprofen and Tylenol.

When you do make the commitment to start, start slow. I urge you not to allow yourself to become overwhelmed and succumb to nutritional ignorance by giving up. Healthcare professionals and mainstream folks are quick to label individuals like you and I as 'health nuts' because we choose to read labels and make an effort to eat consciously. However, the real food faddist is the inadequate eater that chooses to live on empty calorie (non)foods out of convenience and laziness.

One of the things I am most proud of as I go through this journey is the fact that I am able to support my family's health in a holistic way. In doing this, I am also supporting their mind and spirit by instilling in them a love and respect for their bodies and nature. This is a priority for me, as it is my heartfelt desire that my children pass on these valuable tools for healing down to their children. I hope you join me in this quest. Our children are the future; for it is through them, that we will experience the change we so desperately need!

Chapter 5
Herbs and Your Body

The word 'healing' has its roots in the Greek language and comes from the word 'whole' and 'holistic'. Whether we are focused on being healthy, restoring our health, or moving into a greater level of health, the whole of the being, physical, mental and spiritual, is involved in this process. Holistic medicine deals with the 'whole' person; it treats the body as a whole and integrated system, not as a collection of isolated parts.

Unlike western medicine, herbal medicine recognizes that herbs work synergistically, not just on specific body parts. Medicine can only be truly holistic if it acknowledges the entire being; its patterns of thought, behavior, work and culture, in an effort to understand the source of the dis-ease in the first place. When we acknowledge this, our emphasis shifts towards education, self-care and the promotion of a healthier lifestyle.

Herbs have been successfully used to support health and wholeness, allowing an individual to stay at the peak of vitality and thus prevent dis-ease from developing. They can also be used safely for the alleviation of illness and even the reversal of dis-ease in every system of the body. Herbs are effective in addressing issues affecting the nervous system, the endocrine system, the digestive system, the respiratory system, the lymphatic system, the female and male reproductive systems, the skin, the skeletal system, the glandular system and the urinary system. Providing a detailed and specific breakdown of how these body systems react when under stress and how to identify patterns of dis-ease is beyond the intended scope of this book. However, it should be clear that all of our body's systems are affected even when only one is showing signs of distress. As you embark on this road to healing naturally, you will also learn how to become familiar with your body's signals for dis-ease so that you are able to discern when something is off balance.

For anyone interested in herbs for detoxification, building the immune system and finding relief from certain symptoms, the plant kingdom provides abundantly. There are herbs that act as herbal foods in nurturing our wholeness and well being. These tonic herbs play an important and integral part in the maintenance of health.

From my experience, the simplest way to approach the usage of herbs is to categorize them by looking at what kinds of problems they can help alleviate. Herbal properties can be divided into three main categories according to the actions they generate in the body. They are as follows:

1. Detoxification and elimination
2. Support for the body's immune system
3. Symptom relieving

To take it a step further, within those three categories there are also corresponding properties, and some herbs are known to have properties that fall under all three categories. I know this can be overwhelming and confusing to grasp at first, and it is not necessary for you to remember all of it at this point. However, it will be important for you to become familiar with the herbal properties and terms if your focus will be to help others outside of your immediate family. In order to keep things simple and stay within the scope of this book, I will focus on giving you brief explanations for the three main categories, as well as some of the corresponding properties.

1.   Herbs Used for Detoxification and Elimination.   These herbs are typically used when the body has accumulated so much toxicity that it needs to be flushed out.   Cleansing herbs have different properties that influence different parts of the body while still working synergistically. Safe cleansing herbs tend to support the body's natural process. An example would be of herbs with laxative properties like <u>Yellow Dock</u> and <u>Dandelion Root</u>, which clean the bowels, while herbs with alternative properties such as <u>Nettles</u> and <u>Cleavers</u>, would gently cleanse the blood.

2.   Herbs Used for Building and Toning. Tonics are herbs that strengthen the body and as a result improve the function of the internal organs. They either strengthen or enliven a specific organ or the whole body, particularly when taken over an extended period

of time. Tonics are typically very gentle and have a mild but profound effect on the body. Tonics may also be used specifically to ward off a known health problem or a family weakness. Some examples of common gentle tonics are <u>Garlic</u>, <u>Echinacea</u>, <u>St. John's Wort</u> and <u>Nettles</u>.

3.   Herbs Used to Relieve Symptoms. These herbs counteract or relieve specific symptoms. It is good to note that there are herbs whose physiological impact makes them especially effective for supporting the different pathways of elimination in the body. As a general example, if you were dealing with spasms, you would use an antispasmodic herb. If you were dealing with an infection, then you would employ the use of an herb with antibiotic properties.

- o   For the digestive system and colon use a laxative
- o   For the kidneys and urinary system use a diuretic
- o   For the liver and blood use a hepatic, alternative
- o   For the lymphatic system use an alternative, lymphatic, tonic
- o   For skin use a diaphoretic, alternative
- o   For the respiratory system use an expectorant, anti-catarrhal
- o   For systemic support in general use a tonic, alternative, adaptogen, anti-microbial

You will note that the above examples do not specify a particular herb or even mention a remedy; that will be your challenge to discern, as you continue gaining knowledge.

4.   Contraindications. Although herbs are generally safe to use, it is important to become aware of a particular herb's specific action so that you may be in a position to determine if caution is needed, before administering it, whether it is for yourself or a family member.

For example, pregnant women respond differently to certain herbs, even when given in small doses. More specifically, there are certain herbs that serve to stimulate the uterus. These herbs are called Emmenagogues. In a non-pregnant state, Emmenagogues are of no consequence; however, these should be avoided during pregnancy as they may cause stimulation and spasms in the uterus, which may trigger a miscarriage. It should also be noted that there are also certain herbs that are known to have a positive toning effect on the uterus during pregnancy. These tonic herbs strengthen the uterus, alleviate morning sickness, prevent hemorrhaging after birth, provide an energy boost, reduce pain during labor, etc. Some of these amazing herbs are mentioned on *Page 44*.

Herbs that have a diuretic action, like Parsley, should not be given to pregnant women in medicinal doses. Additionally, individuals that have a very nervous disposition may require less of an herb that is a known stimulant.

Although not very common, there are individuals that may have an allergic reaction to certain herbs. You should immediately discontinue any remedy, if you notice a skin rash, diarrhea, or anything out of the ordinary. Individuals with high blood pressure should obviously avoid herbs that stimulate the heart or constrict blood capillaries.

As you expand on this journey, it would be good for you to get into the habit of researching all of the herbs you use (including those mentioned in any formula shared in this book) for any contraindications. If you have any doubt on a particular herb's action, research it until you find an answer. If you do not find the answers with the resources available to you, then do without it. This is another reason why having one or more good herbal reference books available in your home personal library will become vital.

Acute vs. Chronic Illness:

It is important to know the difference between acute and chronic illness. Generally speaking, acute health issues are short term; they come quickly and aggressively and respond well to treatment. (Ex: Fevers, headaches, cuts, wounds, insect bites, stomach issues, menstrual cramps, burns, etc.) Herbal remedies work very well for acute situations, BUT they don't always have a dramatic or immediate effect as you would expect to receive when using pharmaceutical drug. They take time. This is where your diet, your body's condition, and its overall ability to heal will play a role in how you respond to a remedy.

Chapter 6
Herbal Classifications and Corresponding Properties

You will quickly discover that there exists an overwhelming variety of herbs and that they each have many different functions. They may act in general to support the system as a whole, or be very specific in targeting a particular illness. Just remember that herbs are chosen to suit the individual and the way in which disease manifests itself in that individual. Therefore, one size does not fit all. This diversity and abundance is the beauty and joy of herbalism. Ironically, it is also the frustration of every herbalist!

Detoxifying Herbs	Building and Toning Herbs	Symptom Relieving Herbs
Alternatives	Aphrodisiacs	Anodynes
Anthelmintics	Astringents	Antacids
Anticatarrhals	Cardiacs	Antibiotics
Aperients	Diaphoretics	Antiemetics
Cathartics	Emmenagogues	Antipyretics
Cholagogues	Galactagogues	Antipasmodics
Deobstruents	Hepatics	Aromatics
Discutients	Nervines	Carminatives
Diuretics	Nutritives	Condiments
Emetics	Oxytocics	Demulcents
Expectorants	Stomachics	Diaphoretics
Laxatives	Tonics	Emetics
Lithotriptics	Vulneraries	Emmenagogues
Lymphatics		Emollients
Parasiticides		Febrifuges
Purgatives		Hemostatics
		Mucilages
		Oxytocics
		Rubefacients
		Sedatives
		Sialagogues
		Stimulants
		Styptics

Below is an illustration showing where certain common herbs can help. These are by no means the only ones. Getting to know your herbs and experimenting with them is all part of the learning process.

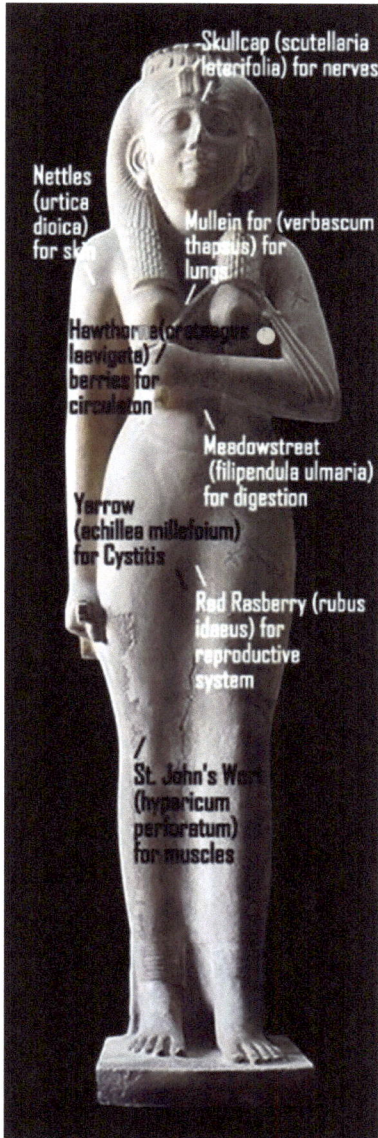

Skullcap (scutellaria leterifolia) for nerves

Nettles (urtica dioica) for skin

Mullein for (verbascum thapsus) for lungs

Hawthorne (crataegus laevigata) berries for circulation

Meadowstreet (filipendula ulmaria) for digestion

Yarrow (achillea millefolium) for Cystitis

Red Rasberry (rubus idaeus) for reproductive system

St. John's Wort (hyparicum perforatum) for muscles

Herbs That Should Be Avoided During Pregnancy:

These herbs will not always act as abortifacients; however, it is prudent to avoid them if you know you are pregnant.

Angelica, Autumn Crocus
Barberry, Basil, Black Cohosh, Blue Cohosh, Blue Vervain, Buckthorn
Calendula, Camphor, Caraway Seed, Cascara Sagrada, Castor oil, Catnip, Celery Seed, Chamomile
Dong Quai
Ephedra
False Unicorn, Feverfew, Flax Seed
Gentian Root, Ginger, Ginseng, Golden Seal
Hops, Horseradish (fresh), Hyssop
Juniper
Larkspur, Lavender
Male Fern, Mandrake, Marjoram, Marshmallow, Mistletoe, Motherwort, Mugwort
Origanum, Osha Root
Pennyroyal, Poke Root
Rosemary (in flower), Rue
Saffron Stigmas, Sage, Senna, Southernwood, Sumac Berries
Tansy, Thuja, Thyme, Turkey Rhubarb
Wormwood

Beneficial Herbs for Pregnancy:

Alfalfa Leaf – Builds red blood cells and promotes lactation.

Comfrey – Provides the needed vitamins and minerals for preventing backaches as well as the amino acids needed for strong abdominals and healthy babies. Helps prevent hemorrhage.

Dandelion Leaf – High in Potassium provides the needed Folic Acid to help prevent health defects.

Lamb's Quarters – Provides the needed Folic Acid to help prevent health defects.

Nettle leaf – High in Vit A, C, D, K, Calcium, Iron, Potassium, aids kidneys, nourishes mother and baby, eases leg cramps, prevents hemorrhage, and reduces hemorrhoids.

Parsley (fresh) – High in Vit C, provides the needed Folic Acid to aid in preventing health defects. Do not use in medicinal doses during pregnancy.

Red Raspberry Leaf – Rich in Vit A, B C, E, Calcium, Iron, tones uterus, helps prevent miscarriage and hemorrhage, eases morning sickness, reduces labor pain, helps with the after birth, increases milk production.

Yellow Dock Root – Prevents anemia. Large doses are not recommended over a long period.

Herbal Index for Your Easy Reference

Abscess:
Cleavers, Echinacea, Garlic, Golden Seal, Lobelia, Marshmallow, Myrrh

Acne:
Burdock root, Chamomile, Cleavers, Dandelion, Echinacea, Garlic, Prickly Ash, Sarsaparilla, Yellow Dock

Anxiety:
Chamomile, St. John's Wort, Skullcap, Valerian, Balm, Hyssop, Oats, Peppermint

Appendicitis:
Golden Seal, Wild Yam

Appetite Loss:
Blessed Thistle, Chamomile, Golden Seal

Arthritis:
Celery seed, Prickly Ash, Wild Yam, Juniper, Wintergreen, Yarrow

Asthma:
Elecampane, Black Haw, Blood Root, Coltsfoot, Hops, Mullein, Sundew, Wild Cherry Bark

Blood Pressure (High):
Hawthorn, Yarrow, Balm, Black Haw, Cramp Bark, Yarrow

Boils:
Echinacea, Garlic, Poke Root, Chickweed, Cleavers, Coltsfoot, Comfrey, Fenugreek, Flax Seed, Plantain, Marshmallow

Bronchitis:
Blood Root, Coltsfoot, Echinacea, Elecampane, Garlic, Mullein, Comfrey, Fennel, Fenugreek, Flax Seed, Plantain, Hyssop, Marshmallow, Thyme

Bruises:
Arnica, Elder, Chickweed, Marigold, St. John's Wort

Burns:
Aloe, Elder, Marigold, Plantain, St. John's Wort, Chamomile, Chickweed, Comfrey

Circulation:
Cayenne, Ginger, Prickly Ash, Rosemary

Colds:
Cayenne, Elder, Echinacea, Garlic, Ginger, Golden Rod, Golden Seal, Hyssop, Peppermint, Yarrow

Colic:
Angelica, Ginger, Peppermint, Valerian, Allspice, Anise seed, Chamomile

Colitis:
Agrimony, Bayberry, Comfrey, Marshmallow, Meadowstreet

Conjunctivitis:
Chamomile, Golden Seal, Marigold, Fennel

Constipation:
Buckthorn, Cascara Sagrada, Rhubarb Root, Senna, Yellow Dock, Aloe, Figwort, Flax Seed, Licorice

Cough:
Angelica, Aniseed Coltsfoot, Comfrey, Elecampane, Garlic, Golden Seal, Hyssop, Mullein, Plantain, Marshmallow, Thyme

Cramps:
Black Cohosh, Cramp Bark, Skullcap, Valerian, Wild Yam, Cayenne, Ginger

Cystitis:
Couchgrass, Echinacea, Juniper, Yarrow, Cleavers, Corn Silk

Depression:
Damiana, Oats, Skullcap, Wormwood, Balm, Celery, Chamomile, Mugwort, Rosemary, Valerian

Diarrhea:
Agrimony, Bayberry, Comfrey, Meadowstreet, Plantain, Blessed Thistle,

Diverticulitis:
Wild Yam, Comfrey, Chamomile, Marshmallow

Earache:
Chamomile, Hyssop, Mullein, Pennywort

Eczema:
Burdock, Chickweed, Cleavers, Figwort, Golden Seal, Nettles

Epilepsy:
Hyssop, Skullcap, Passion Flower, Valerian

Fever:
Blue Vervain, Boneset, Catnip, Cayenne, Cinnamon, Cloves, Ginger, Chamomile, Peppermint, Red Raspberry

Flatulence:
Angelica, Cayenne, Fennel, Ginger, Aniseed, Balm, Blessed Thistle, Catnip, Chamomile, Cloves, Horseradish, Juniper, Mugwort, Parsley, Peppermint, Thyme, Valerian, Wormwood

Fungus Infection:
Celandine, Golden Seal, Marigold, Myrrh, Pau d'arco

Gall-Bladder:
Dandelion, Milk Thistle, Vervain, Wild Yam, Golden Seal, Celandine, Marigold

Gastritis:
Comfrey, Golden Seal, Marshmallow, Meadowstreet, Slippery Elm, Chamomile, Irish Moss, Licorice

Gingivitis:
Echinacea, Golden Seal, Oak Bark, Poke Root, Bayberry, Garlic, Vervain

Glands:
Cleavers, Echinacea, Garlic, Ginger, Ginseng, Kelp, Licorice Root, Lobelia, Mullein, Marigold, Poke Root

Hayfever:
Golden Seal, Elder, Garlic, Peppermint

Heartburn:
Comfrey, Marshmallow, Meadowstreet, Irish Moss, Rosemary, Skullcap, Slippery Elm, Wormwood, Yarrow

Hemorrhoids:
Lady's Mantle, Comfrey, Plantain, Oak

Indigestion:
Balm, Cayenne, Chamomile, Fennel, Ginger, Peppermint, Valerian, Wild Yam, Wormwood, Allspice, Blessed Thistle, Catnip, Cloves, Dill, Mugwort, Rosemary, Thyme

Infection:
Cleavers, Echinacea, Garlic, Golden Seal, Myrrh, Cayenne, Fenugreek, Ginger, Thyme, Wormwood

Influenza:
Cayenne, Echinacea, Elder, Garlic, Ginger, Golden Seal, Peppermint, Pleurisy Root,

Insomnia:
Hops, Passion Flower, Valerian, Wild Lettuce, Chamomile, Skullcap

Itching:
Chickweed, Golden Seal, Marigold, Chamomile, Cleavers, Peppermint, St. John's Wort

Kidney Stones:
Corn Silk, Couchgrass, Dandelion, Gravel Root, Parsley, Plantain, Spearmint, Yarrow

Labor Pains:
Black Cohosh, Cramp Bark, Motherwort, Wild Yam, Blue Cohosh, Valerian, Wild Lettuce

Laryngitis:
Echinacea, Golden Seal, Oak, Thyme, Cayenne, Chamomile, Fenugreek, Golden Rod, Poke Root

Liver:
Black Root, Dandelion, Yellow Dock, Burdock, Garlic, Golden Seal, Wild Yam

Menopause:
Black Cohosh, Chaste Tree, False Unicorn Root, Golden Seal, St. John's Wort

Menstruation:
(Delayed)
Blue Cohosh, Chaste Tree, False Unicorn Root, Parsley, Wormwood, Marigold, Motherwort, Mugwort, Yarrow

Menstruation:
(Excessive)
Periwinkle, Golden Seal, Lady's Mantle

Menstruation:
(Painful)
Black Cohosh, Black Haw, Cramp Bark, St. John's Wort, Skullcap, Valerian, Wild Lettuce, Chaste Tree, False Unicorn Root, Marigold, Wild Yam

Migraine:
Feverfew, Peppermint, Skullcap, Wormwood

Mouth Ulcers:
Myrrh, Red Sage, Chamomile, Lady's Mantle, Oak

Nausea:
Chamomile, Meadowstreet, Peppermint, Cayenne, Cinnamon, Cloves, Fennel

Stress:
Damiana, St. John's Wort, Skullcap, Balm, Chamomile, Hops, Oats, Passion Flower, Valerian, Wild Lettuce, Wormwood

Nosebleed:
Lady's Mantle, Marigold

Ovarian Pain:
Valerian, Passion Flower, St. John's Wort, Skullcap, Wild Yam

Pain:
Black Cohosh, Valerian, Wild Lettuce, Cramp Bark, Hops, Rosemary, Skullcap

Palpitations:
Motherwort, Skullcap, Valerian

Pregnancy Tonic:
Alfalfa, Comfrey, Nettle, Raspberry Leaf, Squaw Vine

Pre-Menstrual Tension:
Calendula, Chaste Tree, Skullcap, Valerian

Prostate:
Damiana, Horsetail, Saw Palmetto, Hydrangea, Corn Silk, Couchgrass

Psoriasis:
Burdock, Cleavers, Figwort, Red Clover, Sarsaparilla, Yellow Dock, Chickweed, Flax Seed, Sassafras

Rheumatism:
Angelica, Black Cohosh, Prickly Ash, Wild Lettuce, Wild Yam, Wintergreen, Yarrow, Burdock, Dandelion, Elder, Cayenne, Horsetail, St. John's Wort

Sciatica:
Black Cohosh, St. John's Wort, Yarrow

Shingles:
Passion Flower, St. John's Wort, Flax Seed, Hops, Skullcap, Valerian, Wild Lettuce, Wild Yam

Sinusitis:
Elder, Garlic, Golden Rod, Golden Seal, Poke Root, Chamomile, Peppermint, Thyme, Yarrow

Tension:
Motherwort, Passion Flower, St. John's Wort, Skullcap, Valerian, Vervain, Wild Lettuce, Balm, Damiana, Hops

Tonsillitis:
Cleavers, Echinacea, Garlic, Golden Seal, Myrrh, Poke Root, Red Sage, Thyme

Travel Sickness:
Peppermint

Tumors:
Cleavers, Comfrey, Elder, Fenugreek, Red Clover, Thuja

Ulcers:
Comfrey, Marshmallow, Meadowstreet, Slippery Elm, Golden Seal, Irish Moss, Licorice

Varicose Veins:
Hawthorn, St. John's Wort

Vomiting:
Meadowstreet, Cinnamon, Cloves, Comfrey, False Unicorn Root, Peppermint, Rosemary

Water Retention:
Dandelion, Gravel Root, Juniper s, Celery Seed, Corn Silk, Horsetail, Parsley, Yarrow

Whooping Cough:
Coltsfoot, Black Cohosh, Garlic, Mullein, Pansy, Red Clover

Worms:
Garlic, Quassia, Tansy, Black Walnut, Wormwood

Wounds:
Chickweed, Comfrey, Elder, Golden Seal, Plantain, St. John's Wort, Garlic, Marshmallow, Fenugreek

Chapter 7
Herbs You Should Get To Know

All of the medicinal plants described in this section are safe and nontoxic, with few if any negative side effects. That is the beauty of herbal medicine! These are the most commonly known herbs, which are easily found in your yard, the wild, or could be grown in your home garden.

Aloe Vera (aloe barbadensis)

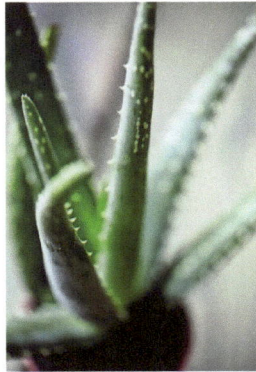

Aloe is probably one of the most commonly known household herbal plants around today. It has historically been known for assisting the function of the gastrointestinal tract, and for its properties of soothing, cleansing and helping the body maintain healthy tissues. This plant has a reputation for facilitating digestion, aiding blood and lymphatic circulation, as well as kidney, liver and gall bladder functions. It has been used internally where a powerful cathartic is needed. In small dosage, it is said to increase the menstrual flow. Externally, the juice is used fresh for minor burns, sunburn, and insect bites.

Herbal Actions: Cathartic, vulnerary, emmenagogue, vermifuge, hepatic, demulcent.
Parts Typically Used: Solidified gel from the leaves
Effective Combinations: If used internally to increase menstrual flow, it should be combined with carminatives to reduce griping.
Growing Zone(s): Indoors in zones 9-11

Basil (ocimum basilicum)

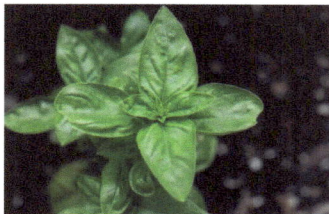

Basil is well regarded in the culinary world for its distinctive flavor and scent. It is valued even more by healers for its medicinal properties. This "royal" herb is said to benefit the digestive and nervous systems, easing gas and stomach cramps and relieving nausea and vomiting. It has mild sedative properties and has been found to be very helpful when dealing with nervous irritability and fatigue, depression, anxiety, and insomnia. Its antibacterial properties make it excellent for use in insect bites, stings, for parasites and skin disorders. Basil also guards the body against free radical damage, while protecting cells and chromosomes from radiation damage.

Herbal Actions: Antioxidant, antibiotic, anti-inflammatory, anti-bacterial
Parts typically used: Leaf and flowering top
Used in: Infusion, juice, tincture, external
Growing Zone(s): Annual (indoors and outdoors)

Burdock *(arctium lappa)*

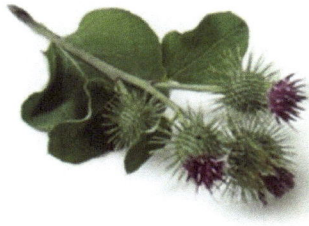

Burdock is quite valuable in its healing properties for the treatment of a multitude of skin conditions and dandruff. It may be most effective for psoriasis if used over a prolonged period of time. All types of eczema can be dealt with effectively with the prolonged use of Burdock. It is a natural blood purifier and detoxifier. Part of the action of this herb is through the bitter stimulation of the digestive juices and especially of bile secretion. As a result, it will also aid digestion and appetite. Externally, it helps to speed up the healing of wounds and ulcers.

Herbal Actions: Alterative, diuretic, bitter, laxative, tonic, vulnerary.
Parts typically used: Roots and rhizome harvested in Fall
Often Used in: decoction, tincture
Growing Zone(s): 2-10

Cayenne *(capsicum annum)*

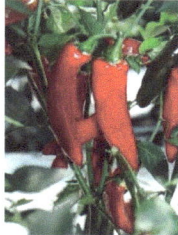

If you set out to master at least one herb, master Cayenne! It is one of the most useful herbs available to man today. It is known to regulate blood flow, equalizing and strengthening the heart, arteries, capillaries, and nerves. It serves as a wonderful tonic and is specific for the circulatory and digestive system. It is used to aid circulation (cold hands and feet), ward off colds, sore throats, laryngitis, flatulence, balance blood pressure levels, and resist abnormal bleeding. Externally it said to be useful for rheumatic pain and to relieve shingles.

Herbal Actions: Stimulant, carminative, tonic, sialagogue, rubefacient, anti-catarrhal, anti-emetic, anti-microbial, diaphoretic.
Parts typically used: Fruit
Used in: Infusions, tinctures, ointments
Growing Zone(s): 9-11

Chamomile *(chamaemelum nobile)*

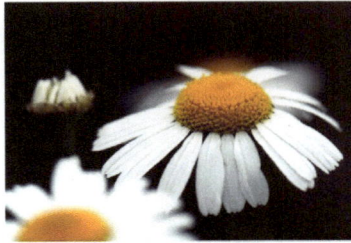

Chamomile is one of my favorite herbs. It is extremely gentle and safe to use with children. Coveted for its sedative properties, it will contribute its relaxing actions in any combination and is commonly used when dealing with anxiety and insomnia. It is often used for gastritis, inflammations, indigestion, sore throats, muscle spasms, infections, nasal catarrh and as an effective eye wash for sore eyes. Chamomile nourishes the respiratory tract and helps alleviate discomfort associated with the menstrual cycle.

Herbal Action: Anti-spasmodic, carminative, anti-inflammatory, analgesic, antiseptic, vulnerary, aromatic, bitter, diaphoretic, emmenagogue, nervine, sedative, tonic
Parts typically used: Flowers and leaves harvested in Spring and Summer
Used in: Infusions, tinctures
Growing Zone(s): 5-8

Chickweed (stellaria media)

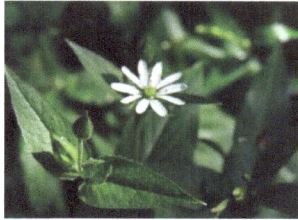

Chickweed has a long standing reputation for being useful when dealing with skin issues such as eczema, skin rashes, skin sores, boils and abscesses. It helps the body eliminate mucus and fatty plaque from the system and it is a natural blood cleanser. Chickweed is an excellent choice for relieving muscular rheumatism and urinary tract inflammations. It can also soothe minor burns and be used to draw out thorns and splinters. You might be surprised to know that this humble herb is also high in calcium, iron, magnesium, manganese, selenium, silica, sodium, phosphorus, potassium, zinc, Vitamins A, B-1, B-2, and C. Since it is abundant on our farm, we often enjoy it as a snack as well as use it in our salads.

Herbal Actions: Astringent, antirheumatic, demulcent, emollient, mild laxative
Parts typically used: Aerial pars harvested in Spring, Summer, Fall, and Winter
Used in: Infusion, external
Growing Zone(s): 7

Cleavers (*gallium aparine*)

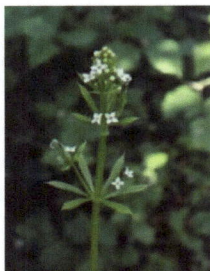

Cleavers are quite possibly the best tonic for the lymphatic system. It has alternative and diuretic actions, which makes it ideal for swollen glands, tonsillitis, and adenoids. It is widely used in skin conditions such as psoriasis. It is also very useful in the dealing with cystitis and other urinary conditions where there is pain. There is a long tradition of its use with ulcers and tumors, which may be the result of lymphatic drainage.

Herbal Actions: Diuretic, alternative, anti-inflammatory, tonic, astringent, anti-neoplastic, hepatic, laxative, vulnerary
Parts typically used: Dried aerial parts and the fresh expressed juice harvested in Spring
Used in: Infusion, tincture
Growing Zone(s): 5-6

Comfrey (symphytum officinale)

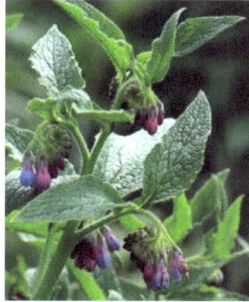

Comfrey is considered one of nature's greatest healers. It is a powerful herb that nourishes the pituitary gland (the master gland of the body). Comfrey has been used to help with broken bones and it is known to speed up wound healing and guard against scar tissue. It has also been used in dealing with arthritic joints, sprains, bruises and other traumatic injuries. No other herb is quite as effective when used for skin conditions such as sores, diaper rash, acne, and psoriasis. It is also helpful with varicose ulcers and hemorrhoids.

Herbal Actions: Vulnerary, demulcent, astringent, expectorant, emollient, pectoral, tonic, anti-inflammatory
Parts typically used: Root and rhizome, leaf harvested in Spring
Used in: External- ointment, poultice, compress, oil
Growing Zone(s: 3-8

Dandelion (taraxacum officinale)

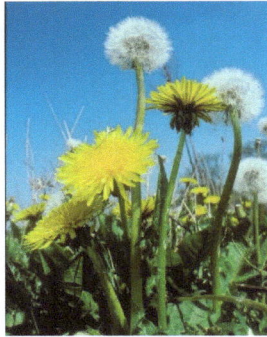

Dandelion in my opinion is the most widely disrespected super herb on the planet. It is no coincidence that the most effective liver detox medicine grows in virtually every yard in America. Dandelion is a very powerful diuretic and liver tonic, as it aids any inflammation and congestion of the liver and gall bladder. It is also quite effective with rheumatism, acne, psoriasis, where liver stimulation and detoxification is needed. It is rich in potassium, which helps balance the body.

Herbal Actions: Diuretic, cholagogue, anti-rheumatic, laxative, tonic, anti-bilious, hepatic
Parts typically used: Leaf harvested in Spring, Summer, Fall and Winter, root harvested in Summer
Used in: Decoction, infusion, tincture, juice
Growing Zone(s): 3-10

Echinacea *(echinacea angustifolia)*

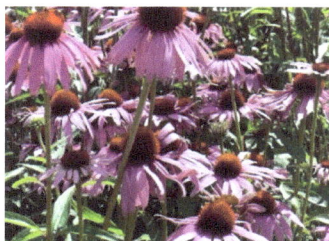

Echinacea is one of the most effective herbs available to rid the body of microbial, viral, and bacterial infections. It has been successfully used in conditions such as boils, and septicemia. It is highly useful for upper respiratory tract infections such as tonsillitis, laryngitis, catarrh. Externally, it may be used for sores, cuts and insect bites.

Herbal Actions: Anti-microbial, alternative, anti-catarrhal, tonic
Parts typically used: Cone flower, roots harvested in Fall
Used in: Decoction, tincture
Growing Zone(s): 3-10

Elder (sambucus nigra)

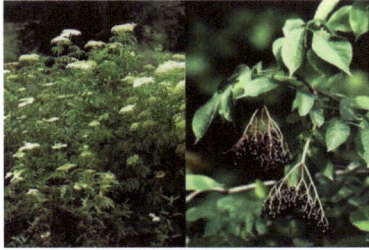

The Elder plant is often called a complete medicine chest when one considers that the root, bark, leaves and berries are all effectively used in healing. The leaves are used for wounds, bruises, sprains and chilblains. The flowers and berries are more commonly used in cordials for colds and influenza where catarrhal inflammation of the upper respiratory tract is an issue.

Herbal Actions: Bark: purgative, emetic, diuretic; Leaves: Externally emollient and vulnerary, internally as purgative, expectorant, diuretic and diaphoretic; Flowers: diaphoretic, anti-catarrhal, pectoral; Berries: diaphoretic, diuretic, laxative
Parts typically used: Bark, flowers, berries, leaves harvested in Summer and Fall
Used in: Infusion, juice, ointment, tincture
Growing Zone(s):4-7

Garlic *(allium sativum)*

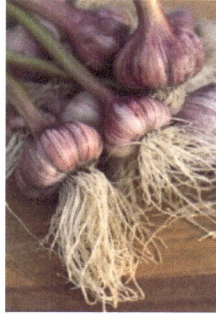

Garlic is among the few herbs that have universal usage and recognition. When taken daily it is known to aid and support the body in ways that no other herb can. It is one of the most effective anti-microbial plants available, acting on bacteria, viruses and alimentary parasites. It is used for respiratory infections such as chronic bronchitis, catarrh, recurrent colds and influenza. It may also be used as a preventative for most infectious conditions, digestive as well as respiratory. In addition, it will reduce blood pressure and blood cholesterol levels, when taken over a period of time. It has been used externally for ringworm.

Herbal Actions: Antiseptic, anti-microbial, diaphoretic, cholagogue, hypotensive, anti-spasmodic, alternative, anthelmintic, anti-catarrhal, carminative, expectorant, pectoral, rubefacient, stimulant, tonic, vulnerary.
Parts typically used: Bulb harvested in Fall
Growing Zone(s):7-9

Ginger *(zingiber officinale)*

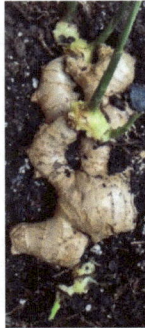

Although it is highly coveted as a culinary herb, its superb medicinal properties cannot be ignored. It contains a proteolytic enzyme that has been shown to reduce inflammation and help repair damaged joints and cartilage tissue. It is a favorite for arthritis and joint pain, gastrointestinal infections, food poisoning, poor circulation, colds, flu, respiratory congestion and sore throat. It is known to improve circulation in the pelvis and this makes it effective in reproductive tonics (for men and women), as well as for menstrual cramps and PMS. Several studies have confirmed how Ginger actually lowers blood-pressure and is more effective for nausea, motion sickness, and morning sickness than over-the counter medications. Ginger is also said to rival anti-nausea drugs for chemotherapy, without the harmful side effects.

Herbal Actions: Stimulant, carminative, rubefacient, diaphoretic, aromatic, emmenagogue, sialgogue
Parts typically used: Rootstock
Used in: Infusion, decoction, tincture, external
Growing Zone(s): 9-12

Golden Seal *(hydrastis canadensis)*

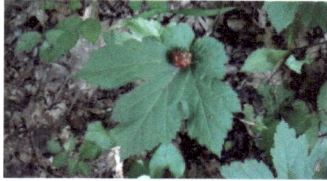

Goldenseal is used both internally and externally to help the body fight infections with its nutritional properties. It helps the body soothe inflammations of the mucous membranes and balance their function. It is especially nourishing to the liver, glandular and respiratory systems. Goldenseal is helpful with most digestive issues a and externally it is used for eczema, ringworm, earaches and conjuvitis.

Herbal Actions: Tonic, astringent, anti-catarrhal, laxative, oxytocic, bitter, alterative, anti-billious, cholagogue, emmenagogue, expectorant, hepatic, pectoral, vulnerary
Parts typically used: Root and rhizome
Used in: Infusion, tincture
Growing Zone(s): 4-7

Hawthorn *(crataegus laevigata)*

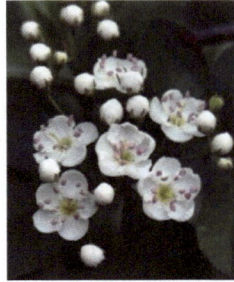

Hawthorn berries are an excellent tonic for the heart and circulatory system. They will move the heart to function normally in a gentle way. As a long-term remedy, it may be used in heart failure or weakness. It can be used in cases of palpitations and as a tonic for the circulatory system when dealing with high blood pressure.

Herbal Actions: Cardiac tonic, hypotensive, diuretic
Parts typically used: Ripe fruits harvested in Fall
Used in: Infusions, tinctures
Growing Zone(s):3-8

Hyssop (hyssopus officinalis)

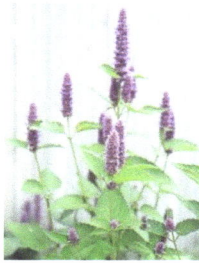

Hyssop has a pretty wide range of uses that are attributed to its anti-spasmodic actions. It is useful with coughs, bronchitis, and chronic catarrh. Its diaphoretic properties make it effective for use with the common cold. As a nervine, it can be used for anxiety, hysteria, and petit mal seizures (a form of epilepsy).

Herbal Actions: Anti-spasmodic, expectorant, diaphoretic, sedative, carminative, anti-catarrhal, aromatic, hepatic, pectoral, tonic, vulnerary
Parts typically used: Dried aerial parts harvested in Summer
Used in: Infusion, tincture
Growing Zone(s): 3-8

Lavender *(lavandula angustifolia)*

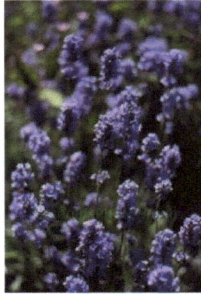

Lavender is an extremely aromatic herb that has many uses. It is quite effective for stress-related headaches. It can be useful with depression, especially when combined with other remedies. It is a gentle tonic to the nervous system, and as such it aids with nervousness and promotes natural sleep. Externally, the oil can be used as a liniment to help ease aches and rheumatism pains.

Herbal Actions: Carminative, anti-spasmodic, anti-depressant, rubefacient, anti-emetic, nervine
Parts typically used: Flowers harvested in Summer and Fall
Used in: Infusions, tinctures
Growing Zone(s): 5-8

Lemon Balm *(melissa officinalis)*

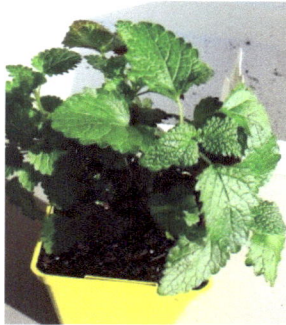

Lemon Balm is one of the most important members of the mint family. Its gentle sedative properties make it an effective aid for depression, stress, anxiety and nervous disorders. It has a tonic effect on the heart and circulatory system, aiding in lowering blood pressure. It can be used in feverish conditions such as the flu. This is one of my favorite herbs for children, as it is known to calm a restless child before bedtime. Lemon Balm has strong anti-viral action and is said to be quite effective against shingles and herpes.

Herbal Actions: Carminative, anti-spasmodic, anti-depressive, diaphoretic, hypotensive, anti-emetic, aromatic, hepatic, nervine, tonic
Parts typically used: Dried aerial parts, or fresh in season
Used in: Infusion, tincture
Growing Zone(s): 5-9

Licorice (glycyrrhiza glabra)

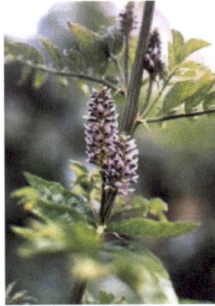

Licorice is quite useful for the endocrine system and for adrenal gland issues. It is widely used for bronchial problems such as catarrh, bronchitis and coughs. It is also used in gastritis, ulcers and for the relief of abdominal colic.

Herbal Actions: Expectorant, demulcent, anti-inflammatory, adrenal agent, anti-spasmodic, mild laxative, emollient, pectoral, tonic
Parts typically used: Dried root
Used in: Decoction, tincture
Growing Zone(s): 7-10

Marigold (calendula officinalis)

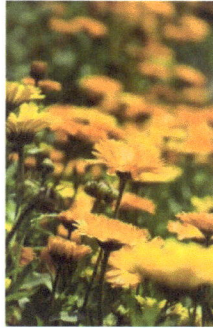

Marigold (also known as Calendula) is one of my preferred herbs to use for inflammation of the skin, external bleeding, bruising or strains. It is ideal for first aid treatment of minor burns and scalds and quite versatile when used as a lotion, poultice or compress. Internally it is said to be effective when used for gastric ulcers, to relieve gall-bladder problems and indigestion. Its antifungal properties help combat infections (internally and externally). It is also useful for delayed or painful menstrual periods.

Herbal Actions: Anti-inflammatory, astringent, vulnerary, anti-microbial, cholagogue, emmenagogue, tonic, anti-bacterial, antispasmodic
Parts typically used: Yellow petals harvested in Summer and Fall
Used in: Infusion, tincture, external
Growing Zone(s): 9-11

Marsh Mallow (althaea officinalis)

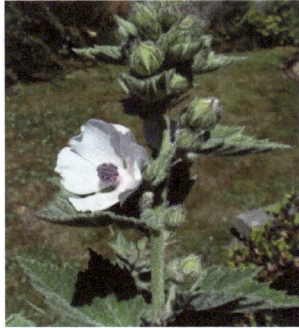

Marshmallow is an excellent demulcent as it contains high mucilage content. The root is typically used for digestive issues and inflammations of the digestive tract and skin. The leaf is often used for the lungs and urinary system. Consider this herb if you are seeking relief from bronchitis, respiratory catarrh and irritating coughs. It is extremely soothing in urethritis and urinary gravel. Externally, the root is indicated in varicose veins and ulcers as well as abscesses and boils.

Herbal Actions: Root – demulcent, diuretic, emollient, vulnerary; leaf – demulcent, expectorant, diuretic, emollient, anti-catarrhal, pectoral.
Parts typically used: Root harvested in Fall and leaf harvested in Spring and Summer
Used in: decoction, infusion, compress, tincture
Growing Zone(s): 3-9

Milk Thistle (silybum marianum)

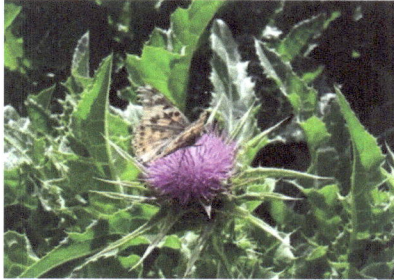

As suggested by its name, Milk Thistle is known in the midwifery world as a safe and effective inducer of breast milk. However, it is likely better known for its liver-protective qualities, as it increases the secretion of bile from the liver and gall-bladder. It is also frequently used with liver disorders and infections.

Herbal Actions: Cholagogue, galactogogue, demulcent, antiviral, anti-depressant, anti-oxidant
Parts typically used: Seeds, leaves and flower heads
Used in: Infusions, tinctures
Growing Zone(s): 5-9

Mullein (verbascum thapsus)

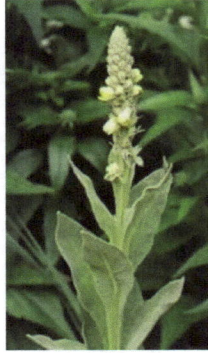

Mullein is a beautiful, exotic looking plant that is an antispasmodic (it relaxes spasms) and an expectorant (it helps expel mucus) herb. Mullein is the go to remedy for spastic coughs, bronchial congestion, chest colds, allergies, and other ailments that involve the respiratory tract as it tones the mucous membranes and stimulates fluid production. The beautiful small yellow flowers contain effective anodynes (relieve pain) with antiseptic infection fighting properties.

Herbal Actions: Expectorant, demulcent, diuretic, sedative, vulnerary, anti-catarrhal, emollient, pectoral, astringent, anti-inflammatory
Parts typically used: Dried leaves and flowers harvested in Summer
Used in: Infusion, tincture, syrup
Growing Zone(s): 4-9

Nettle (*urtica dioica*)

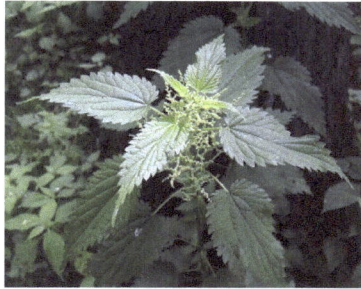

Nettle (also known as "Stinging Nettle") is truly a wonder plant that strengthens and supports the entire body. Rich in vitamins and minerals, it is an excellent tonic herb for bones, joint pain, allergies, liver, prostate, and fertility issues of male and female reproductive systems, menopausal issues. My favorite way of using this lovely herb is in a nourishing tea infusion that fortifies and builds energy levels. The greens are absolutely delicious when steamed with olive oil. The stem and undersides of leaves on the plant have small needle-like protrusions that contain formic acid, the same chemical that causes the pain in bee stings. This acid is destroyed by heating, drying or mashing the harvested leaves. Although I personally find the stings exhilarating and quite therapeutic, I recommend that gloves be worn when harvesting this herb. Several studies have shown the root of this versatile herb to be of value in the relief of benign prostate enlargement. Combine it with Saw Palmetto as a decoction or tincture for best results.

Herbal Actions: Astringent, diuretic, tonic, alternative, rubefacient, hemostatic, galactogogue, hypotensive, anti-allergenic, antiscorbutic
Parts typically used: Aerial parts, root, seed harvested in Spring and Summer
Used in: Infusion, tincture, juice
Growing Zone(s): 3-10

Oats (*avena sativa*)

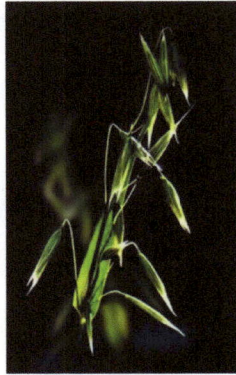

Oats nourish the nervous system when one is under stress. It may be used with other nervines as it is both a relaxant and stimulant, to strengthen the entire nervous system. It is also used in general debility. Oats contain high levels of silic acid in the straw, which explains why it is often used for skin conditions externally.

Herbal Actions: Nervine tonic, anti-depressant, nutritive, demulcent, vulnerary
Parts typically used: Seeds and whole plant harvested in Summer
Used in: Extract, bath, porridge, or oatmeal
Growing Zone(s): 6-7

Parsley (petroselinum crispum)

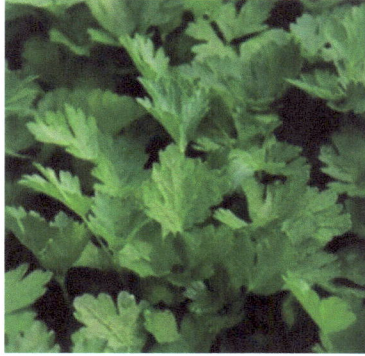

Parsley contains one of the richest sources of Vitamin A, B, C, iron and calcium. It is known to contain more Vitamin C than a single orange! Medicinally speaking, it has three main areas of usage: it is an effective diuretic; building the kidneys and helping the body get rid of excess water. The second area of use is as an emmenagogue, stimulating the menstrual process. The third use is as a carminative, easing flatulence and colic pains that may be associated with it. It also calms and strengthens the nervous system and helps relieve high blood pressure. It is helpful when dealing with jaundice, anemia, adrenal malfunction and low blood sugar. The high chlorophyll content in the leaves has been known to be effective when dealing with cancers.

Herbal Actions: Diuretic, expectorant, emmenagogue, carminative, supposed aphrodisiac, tonic
Parts typically used: Leaves, seeds and root harvested in Summer
Used in: Infusion, tincture
Growing Zone(s): 6-9

Peppermint *(mentha piperata)*

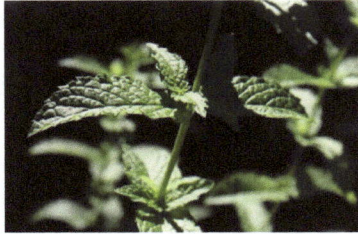

Peppermint is one of my most used herbs. Not only does it have a relaxing effect on the visceral muscles, but it is one of the best carminative agents available to us.   It has anti-flatulent properties and also stimulates bile and digestive juice secretion making it a great aid for intestinal colic, flatulent dyspepsia and related conditions. It acts as a mild anesthetic to the stomach wall, which helps relieve vomiting from pregnancy and travel sickness.

Herbal Actions: Carminative, anti-spasmodic, aromatic, diaphoretic, anti-emetic, nervine, analgesic, anti-catarrhal, anti-microbial, emmenagogue, rubefacient,
stimulant
Parts typically used: Aerial parts
Used in: Tinctures, infusions
Growing Zone(s): 3-7

Plantain *(plantago major)*

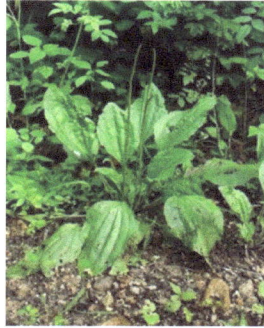

Plantain has so many valuable healing properties. Similar to
Dandelion, it is a super herb that grows like a weed. It is
everywhere! I easily find it on our front lawn, back yard and
everywhere along our farm. It is also visible on highways and by
creeks. Plantain is highly effective in drawing toxins from the body
as it has a long history of use as a blood purifier (for blood
poisoning). Its nutrients enrich the liver and cleanse the blood. It is
also highly effective as a poultice for bug bites, bee stings, boils,
deep infections, and skin disorders. When applied directly to a
wound, it has the ability to help stop bleeding. It is an excellent
wound healer that lessens recovery time. If you are a forager, then
this is the herb for you! It is the perfect emergency food, as it is rich
in vitamins, protein, and starch.

Herbal Actions: Expectorant, demulcent, astringent, diuretic, emollient,
vulnerary
Parts typically used: Seed, root and leaf harvested in Summer and Fall
Used in: Tinctures, infusions, external uses
Growing Zone(s): 3-9

Red Clover *(trifolium pretense)*

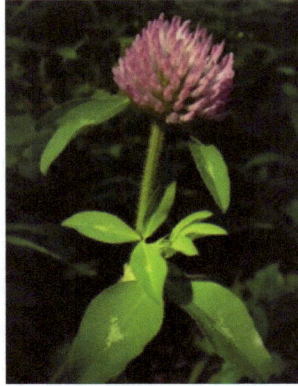

Red Clover became quite popular in the 1930s when it was used with breast cancer, as a blood and lymphatic cleanser. Its expectorant and anti-spasmodic properties make it ideal for use in stubborn coughs, sore throat, bronchitis and whooping cough. It is also helpful for insect bites and stings, mouth ulcers, mood swings, and menopausal symptoms. It is perfectly safe to use in cases of eczema and psoriasis, in children and adults alike.

Herbal Actions: Lymphatic, alternative, expectorant, anti-spasmodic, nervine, sedative, tonic,
Parts typically used: Flower heads harvested in Spring, Summer and Fall
Used in: Infusion, tincture, syrup, fresh herb, external
Growing Zone(s): 5-9

Red Raspberry *(rubus idaeus)*

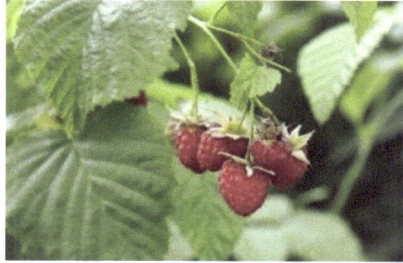

Familiar to most for its tasty fruit, this plant has been used for centuries as an aid to tone and strengthen the womb for childbirth, assisting contractions and helping with any bleeding during labor. It is quite effective if taken regularly during pregnancy and also during labor. Its astringent properties also make it useful when dealing with diarrhea, leucorrhea, mouth ulcers, bleeding gums, inflammations, and fevers.

Herbal Actions: Astringent, tonic, refrigerant, parturient, emmenagogue, febrifuge.
Parts typically used: Leaves and fruit harvested Spring, Summer and Fall
Used in: Infusions, tinctures, external
Growing Zone(s): 4-8

Rosemary *(rosmarinus officinalis)*

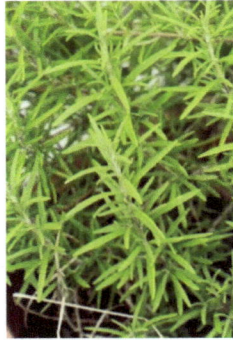

Rosemary is used by most primarily as a culinary herb. However, it has many medicinal properties. It is used as a stimulating tonic and digestive remedy. It acts as a circulatory and nervine stimulant and it is typically used where psychological tension is present. Externally it is used for muscular and arthritic pain, sciatica and neuralgia. It is often used for premature baldness and hair loss, as it also stimulates hair follicles.

Herbal Actions: Carminative, aromatic, anti-spasmodic, anti-depressive, rubefacient, parasiticide, anti-microbial, astringent, emmenagogue, nervine, stimulant
Parts typically used: Leaves and twigs harvested in Summer and Fall
Used in: Infusions, tinctures, external
Growing Zone(s): 8-11

Sage (salvia officinalis)

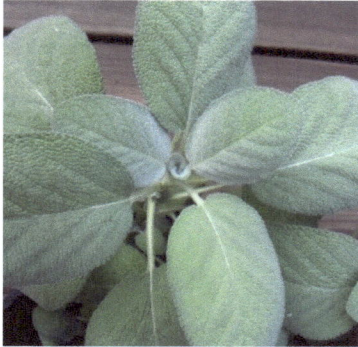

Sage is another culinary gem that is widely used for digestive and menopausal issues, particularly hot flashes. This herb is traditionally associated with longevity. Modern research has shown that it can slow down the progress of Alzheimer's disease. It provides the classic remedy for inflammations of the mouth, gums, tongue, throat and tonsils. When used in a gargle it will help laryngitis and tonsillitis. Red sage is also known to stimulate the muscles of the uterus. It is very effective in dealing with minor cuts and scrapes.

Herbal Actions: Carminative, anti-spasmodic, astringent, antiseptic, uterine stimulant
Parts typically used: Leaves
Used in: Infusion, juice, external
Growing Zone(s): 5-9

Skullcap (scutellaria lateriflora)

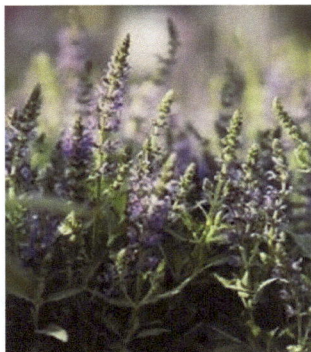

Skullcap (aka Scullcap) is one of the most important nerviness we have available today. It is known to relax extreme states of nervous tension while reviving the central nervous system. It is often used for seizures, epilepsy and depression. And it is also effective as an aid for pre-menstrual tension.

Herbal Actions: Nervine, tonic, sedative, anti-spasmodic, analgesic, hypnotic
Parts typically used: Aerial parts harvested in Summer and Fall
Used in: Infusions, tinctures
Growing Zone(s): 4-8

St. John's Wort (hypericm perfotatum)

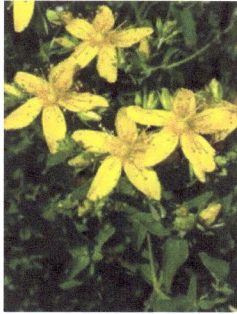

St. John's Wort has amazing sedative and pain reducing properties, which makes it ideal when used for neuralgia, anxiety, tension and related issues. It is especially useful when dealing with menopausal changes that trigger irritability and anxiety. It is commonly used when dealing with depression, but it should be noted that it is slow in action and must be taken for at least a month for one to see the effects. It will ease neuralgic pain, fibrosis, sciatica, and rheumatic pain. St. John's Wort is valuable when used externally for healing and as an anti-inflammatory remedy. When used as a lotion, it speeds up the healing of bruises, wounds, varicose veins, and mild burns. It is also said to have the ability to inhibit the AIDS virus.

Herbal Actions: Anti-inflammatory, astringent, vulnerary, sedative, analgesic
Parts typically used: Aerial parts harvested in Summer and Fall
Used in: Tinctures, infusions, external uses
Growing Zone(s): 4-9

Thyme (thymus vulgaris)

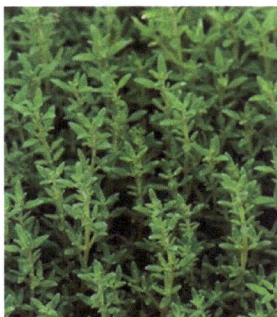

Thyme is frequently used as an expectorant and an antiseptic for the lungs, in order to clear productive coughs and infections. It can also be used for laryngitis, tonsillitis, bronchitis, whooping cough and sore throats, as it is an excellent expectorant. It is effective when used externally for infected wounds and bites. As it is a very gentle astringent, it has found use in diarrhea and bed wetting.

Herbal Actions: Antiseptic, antibiotic, carminative, anti-microbial, anti-spasmodic, expectorant, astringent, anthelmintic, anti-catarrhal, diaphoretic, tonic, vulnerary
Parts typically used: Leaves and flowering tops harvested in Summer
Used in: Infusion, tincture, syrup, external
Growing Zone(s): 4-9

Turmeric (*curcuma longa*)

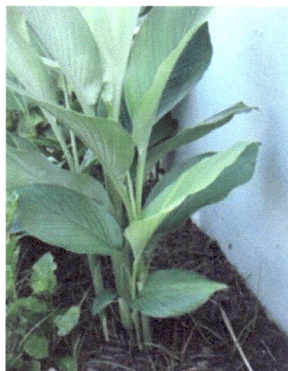

Turmeric has a long history of use in Ayurvedic and Chinese medicine. With long standing use for digestive and liver disorders, it is helpful with nausea, gastritis, excessive stomach acid, indigestion and liver or gall bladder disorders. It is also effective in dealing with menstrual pain, arthritic problems, psoriasis, ringworm or eczema.

Herbal Actions: Carminative, cholagogue, antioxidant, choleretic, detoxifier, antibacterial, anti-inflammatory, hypolipidemic
Parts typically used: Rhizome
Used in: Decoction, ointment, tincture
Growing Zone(s):8-11

Valerian *(valeriana officinalis)*

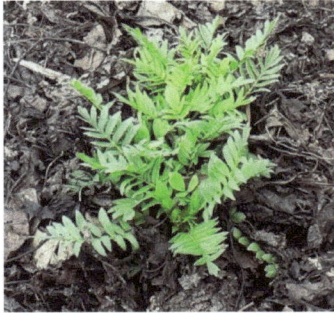

Valerian is considered one of the safest and most useful herbal nerviness available for stress, insomnia, anxiety, over-excitability, and hysterical states. It is effective as a long-term nerve tonic and as a remedy for acute nerve problems, such as headaches and pain. As a tonic, it is recommended in cases of irregular heartbeat and anxiety that affects the heart. It is often used when dealing with high blood pressure. It is also a great reliever of muscle tension, backache, as well as menstrual or muscle cramps.

Herbal Actions: Sedative, hypnotic, anti-spasmodic, hypotensive, carminative, aromatic, nervine, expectorant, analgesic
Parts typically used: Root and rhizome harvested in Fall
Used in: Infusion, tincture, external
Growing Zone(s): 4-9

Yarrow *(achillea millefolium)*

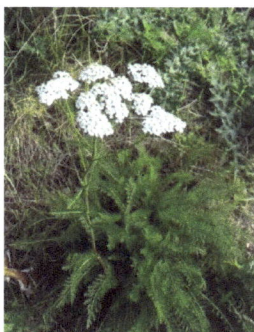

Yarrow is one amazing diaphoretic herb. It is a standard remedy for helping the body deal with fevers. It is known to lower blood pressure, stimulate digestion and tone the blood vessels. As a urinary antiseptic, it is indicated for infections such as cystitis. When used externally it will aid in the healing of wounds. It is considered useful in thrombotic conditions associated with high blood pressure.

Note: The colorful hybrids of Yarrow are bred for aesthetics, rather than for their medicinal properties.

Herbal Actions: Diaphoretic, hypotensive, astringent, diuretic, antiseptic, anti-catarrhal, emmenagogue, hepatic, stimulant, tonic
Parts typically used: Leaves, flowers harvested in Summer and Fall
Used in: Tinctures, infusions
Growing Zone(s):3-9

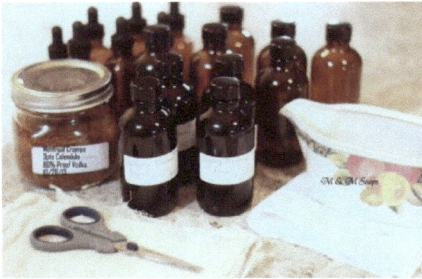

Chapter 8
What You Will Need To Get Started

Before we get into how to prepare certain herbal remedies, it is important that you become aware of a few basic and important guidelines that will help you formulate safe and effective remedies every single time.

1.   Always be sure to use spring or distilled water for any herbal preparation that requires water. **Never** use tap water. I personally prefer spring water over distilled, but either is acceptable. If a remedy requires vinegar, try to source raw apple cider vinegar if possible, as raw cider vinegar will infuse your remedy with additional healing properties. When a certain formula calls for vegetable glycerin, be certain to source "food grade" vegetable glycerin. In addition, when a remedy calls for honey, use raw honey if it is available to you, as raw unpasteurized honey contains many beneficial enzymes that will add another level of healing to your remedy.

2.   The type of containers you use for blending and storing your remedies are very important. Always use glass, ceramic, stainless steel or enamel steel for blending and mixing. NEVER use aluminum, plastic, or iron, as these can react with your preparations, as well as release microscopic amounts of toxic substances. Plastic in particular, releases estrogen, which is harmful to the body. I personally love to use glass Mason jars for blending and curing my herbal formulas. Once a tincture remedy has cured and is ready to be strained from the herbs, I store the final product in a brown glass bottle. The brown bottle is important because it prevents sunlight from further breaking down the

ingredients in my formulas. A frugal alternative to buying brown bottles would be to simply wrap the glass jar containing your finished remedy with a brown paper bag and storing it in a dark cupboard away from sunlight. I also use stainless steel pots when heating is necessary. I will provide a resource for the brown glass bottles in the Resources section of this book found on *Page 120* of this book.

Unused dried herbs should be stored in an airtight container or well-sealed glass jar, away from direct sunlight. When herbs are exposed to heat and sunlight for an extended period of time they become less effective.

3.   Most of the herbal formulas mentioned in this book assume that you will be using <u>dried</u> herbs. Bear in mind however, that if you do choose to use fresh herbs, you must increase your ratio (i.e., double up on the amount used). This is necessary because fresh herbs contain more water than their dried counterparts do. Fresh herbs are generally proportionately less potent for this reason. So for example, if a tincture preparation calls for 3 parts Thyme, you would use 6 parts of fresh Thyme instead. You must also be certain to 'bruise' your fresh herbs to expose the cell membranes and allow for a more effective permeation of your carrier, whether that carrier is going to be oil, water or alcohol. You can easily bruise your herbs in a mortar and pestle using circular grinding motions. I should also mention that it is important to use high quality herbs. If you love gardening, I encourage you to consider growing your own herbs. However, if this is not an option for you, make sure that you get your herbs from reputable sources that specialize in medicinal quality herbs. I will provide you with my favorite herbal resources in the Resources section of this book.

Contraindications:

Although uncommon, some people may be allergic to Chamomile. Itchy eyes, runny nose, and scratchy throat are signs of an allergy. Discontinue its use if these signs manifest.

4.   **<u>Always label your preparations!</u>** No matter what you prepare, even if it is a single herb remedy and you believe you will easily remember, make a label! Trust me, you will not remember. Place a label on your jar including the date it was made, the herbs used in order of significance (i.e., list principal herb

first and end with least significant herb), amount of each herb (i.e., 2 tbsp, 1 cup, etc.), the carrier medium used (i.e., 80% alcohol, glycerin, water) and what the remedy is for and whether it is meant to be used as an external or internal remedy. Get into the habit of keeping notes. I personally have a binder notebook which contains extensive notes on every remedy I formulate, that way I can easily refer to it if I want to keep notes on the results I have experienced or in case I want to tweak the formula in the future. Keeping a journal on your herbal preparations is just a good practice to get into as you increase in your knowledge of herbs. It does not have to be anything fancy. A ruled notebook could serve as your journal, and simple white labels can be used for your jars. Be sure to write neatly so that others in your family can read the remedy as well. <u>This will go a long way in avoiding any mix-ups</u>!

5.   The device you choose to measure your preparations (i.e., scale, spoon, cup, etc.) is also important, because you must keep detailed records in order to be able to determine the strength of your remedy. This will also be useful in the event you want to duplicate the remedy safely or tweak it in the future.

Effective Combinations:

For liver and gall bladder issues, combine Dandelion with Yarrow. If you are suffering from gallstones, only use the <u>root</u> under the supervision of a qualified naturopath.

6.   How and where you store your remedies is important in order to preserve their potency. Avoid storing any of your herbal preparations near light and high heat areas, as heat and light break down substances. A cupboard away from the cooking area or in a basement/cellar is an ideal location. Find your remedies a home in a cool dark place, so that your remedies may enjoy a long shelf-life.

7.   There are times when I have to use the powdered version of certain herbs because that is the only form available to me. You may also experience this along the way. Powdered herbs are sometimes more practical to use, such as when you are making capsules or pills, because using the herb in this form saves you the step of having to grind them into powder form. However, one word of caution if you will be using powdered herbs in tinctures or other

preparations that require a liquid carrier: Powdered herbs tend to settle into a solid clump at the bottom of the jar so just be sure to shake often (once every other day is my rule of thumb). What I do is every time I find myself opening the cupboard they are stored

If you seek to use a specific herb to help with an ailment, you will need to make an herbal infusion, a decoction, a tincture, or capsules.

in, I use that opportunity to give them a good shake.

8.   There are a few basic items, which you will need in order to get started. You will most likely be able to find all of the tools listed here in your kitchen. Here are some of the tools I use the most often when working with herbs:

>   Cheesecloth for straining herbs from liquids
>   A variety of glass jars with lids for storing your herbs, tinctures, salves etc.
>   Mortar and pestle or coffee grinder (to be exclusively used for your herbs)
>   Measuring cups
>   Stainless steel strainer
>   Stainless steel pot with lid

The two ways by which most remedies are administered are internally and externally. Internal methods are ingested through the mouth. External methods are applied to a specific area of the body. In the next chapter, I will get into a few of the most common methods: oxymels, pills, capsules, teas, infusions, decoctions, oils, salves, and tinctures.

If you master these, you will be in a position to address most, if not all of the everyday minor health concerns that may arise with your family. I will provide you with a basic explanation of what these methods are used for and give you simple instructions on how to make them. In the "Herbal Formulas" section of this book, I share with you some of my favorite basic herbal formulas that you can make for your family.

SIMPLER'S METHOD OF MEASURING HERBS

The most versatile and easy system for measuring your herbs is the Simpler's Method because it is based on ratios. Measurements are referred to as "parts". For instance, 3 parts dandelion, 1 part nettle, 2 parts raspberry, is a very common 3:1:2 synergy. This simple way of measuring lets you make your formulation in any volume you wish, whether in ounces, tablespoons, cups, liters, grams etc.

PARTS:
3PARTS PEPPERMINT
1PART NETTLE
2PARTS LAVENDER

PARTS IN TABLESPOONS:
3TABLESPOONS PEPPERMINT
2TABLESPOONS NETTLE
1TABLESPOON LAVENDER

PARTS IN TEASPOONS:
3 TEASPOONS PEPPERMINT
2TEASPOONS NETTLE
1TEASPOON LAVENDER

REMEMBER: THE "PART" IS WHATEVER UNIT OF MEASURE YOU DESIRE (I.E., OUNCE, CUP, TEASPOON, TABLESPOON, ETC).

Chapter 9
Internal Remedies

1.   **OXYMELS**- Oxymels are sweet and sour herbal syrups made of vinegar, honey, and herbs. They are quite pleasant in taste and it is a practical method to employ especially when you are working with a strong tasting herb such as Garlic. These types of remedies are typically used for coughs, throat inflammations, respiratory symptoms, colds and also to soothe the intestinal tract. I love oxymels because both the raw honey and raw apple cider vinegar have amazing healing properties, and they both serve as natural preservatives. One of the benefits of formulating oxymels is that they are so tasty, that even your small children will have no problem taking it. In fact, if they are anything like mine, you might have to hide this remedy from them!

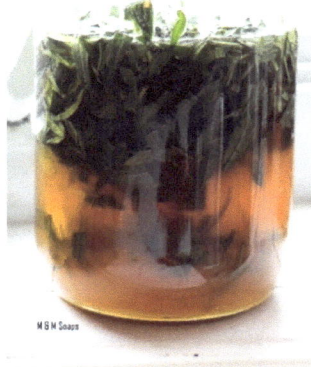

Instructions for Making Oxymels:

(Step 1) Fill a sterilized glass Mason jar half way with your dried herbs. Remember... if you will be using fresh herbs, you must bruise the herb and double the amount!

(Step 2) Now fill the jar to about 1/3 of the way with raw honey. (For a sweeter and thicker oxymels fill the jar half way with honey).

(Step 3) Next fill the jar the rest of the way with raw apple cider vinegar.

(Step 4) Be sure to label your jar with the date, ingredients and what the remedy is for (i.e., cough, cold, etc.). Place in a cool dark place and let sit for 3-4 weeks.

(Step 5) Strain well with a stainless steel strainer or cheesecloth.

(Step 6) Jar once again and label bottle.

Oxymels can be taken in teaspoon to tablespoon measurements. Because of the honey and cider vinegar content, they will keep for a long time but keeping it in the refrigerator will extend its shelf life even more.

2.   **SYRUPS**- Syrups are concentrated herbal decoctions. They are quite pleasant to the palate and are very versatile. The natural benefits of the plant in syrups are aided by sugar or honey, which help to alleviate dry coughs, sore throats, and general irritations of the respiratory system.   Syrups, like oxymels, are preferred by children and the elderly.   They also increase energy levels and nourish the body.

Instructions for Making Syrups:

(Step 1) Take 2 ounces of your herb and place it in a small pot with about 1 quart of filtered or spring water.

(Step 2)   Boil about half of the water away.

(Step 3) Strain and add 2 cups of honey (or maple syrup) or vegetable glycerin to preserve it.

(Step 4) Warm the mixture over low heat, careful not to cook it. You just want to warm it enough to combine the honey or syrup with the herbal liquid.

Sterilize your glass jars or bottles prior to using, by washing them in hot water, drain upside down and place into a cool oven (275°F/140°C) for about 15 minutes.

(Step 5) Remove from heat. At this point you may choose to add a few drops of high quality essential oil like Peppermint.

(Step 6) Pour your syrup into a sterilized glass bottle and label. It may be stored in the refrigerator where it will keep for several weeks.

3.   **CAPSULES**- Herbal capsules are very easy to make. You simply ground your measured and selected herbs very fine and place them into a soluble capsule. You can use a mortar and pestle or electric grinder for this. There are different sizes of capsules ranging from "000" to "5". "00" and "0" are the standard most commonly used sizes. The most commonly used are "00" and "0".

See <u>Page 117</u> for information on each capsule's holding capacity. The density of the herbs you will be working with should be the determining factor in what size capsules you choose. Dipping the capsule in a safe vegetable oil (i.e., non-GMO) right before giving them would assist those that have issues swallowing capsules. When you fill your capsules by hand, you must work quickly as the capsule itself tends to dissolve with body heat if handled for too long. Many herbalists use a handy filling tool, which allows you to make 50 capsules in a fraction of the time. You might want to consider such a tool if you will be making most of your remedies for your family in capsule form. I will provide a link in the Resources section on *Page 120*, for where you may purchase said tool.

4.   **HERBAL PILLS** – One of the advantages of making your own herbal pills, is that you can make them into any size you want for small children and older adults who often have issues taking capsules.

<u>Instructions for Making Herbal Pills</u>:

(Step 1) Follow the same steps as when making capsules, by taking your selected herbs and grinding them into a powder.
(Step 2) Add about 10% of <u>Slippery Elm</u> powder. <u>Slippery Elm</u> is a demulcent and will acts as a binder for your herbal pills. If Slippery Elm is not available, you may also use <u>Comfrey Root.</u>
(Step 3) In a bowl mix your powdered herbs with enough water and raw honey (or maple syrup) to make a sticky paste. Add this gradually, as you want to keep the mixture somewhat firm.
(Step 4) Allow the mixture to sit for a few minutes then roll the mixture into pea-sized balls.

At this point, you can place the pills in a dehydrator to dry. If you do not have a dehydrator, you may place them on a lined cookie sheet inside your oven with just the oven light on. For an even more pleasant experience, roll the pills in carob powder (before drying). Once dried, you should store them in a glass jar in a cool dark place. Remember to label the jar. I find that this is a fun project to do with young children.

5.   **HERBAL TEAS**   - Herbal teas are typically made one or two cups at a time. For practical reasons, I like making a quart or half-gallon jar at a time. Herbal teas are not as potent as infusions and decoctions, but they are extremely valuable beverages to incorporate into your daily routine, as they administer subtle healing energies in small regular doses. Beverage herbal teas should not be confused with medicinal teas (i.e., infusions and decoctions) which require a larger amount of herbs. Herbal teas are a great and healthier substitute for commercial soft drinks and sugary drinks. They keep for about a week when refrigerated and are quite pleasant to drink hot, warm or cold.

ഇൽ

Infusion Tip:

If you want to experience the amazing healing powers of the sun, try making a solar herbal infusion. It is one of my favorite methods for making tea. Solar infusions contain a level of healing that cannot be derived from the conventional method. For a solar infusion, simply place your herbs in a quart glass jar. Fill the jar with cold filtered or spring water and cover tightly. Let the jar sit in direct sunlight for several hours.

ഇൽ

Instructions for Making Herbal Teas:

(Step 1) Place 2-3 tablespoons of your selected herb(s) in a teapot or a sterilized Mason jar.
(Step 2) Bring 16 oz of filtered or spring water to a rolling boil. Pour hot water into teapot or Mason jar. Cover Mason jar. Allow herbs to steep for 15-20 minutes.
(Step 3) Strain and serve.
You may add more water to re-infuse the herbs at least one additional time, but be aware that your second brew will not be as potent.

6.   **HERBAL INFUSIONS** - If you know how to make tea then you can easily make an infusion. Infusions are perhaps the easiest and most preferred method of absorbing the medicinal properties and volatile oils of herbs that are needed for healing. They are typically steeped in hot water so as not to overcook and destroy the beneficial enzymes, vitamins and volatile essential oils in the plant. With some exceptions, they are usually made using the more delicate parts of the plan (i.e., leaves, flowers, buds and berries). A medicinal tea is defined by its potency. For medicinal purposes, the longer you steep the herb, the stronger the tea.

94

Instructions for Making an Herbal Infusion:

(Step 1) Bring a pint of filtered or spring water to a rolling boil.
(Step 2) Add 1 ounce of your dried herb to a glass Mason jar.
(Step 3) Next, add boiling water to jar and cover the jar with its lid to avoid the volatile oils from evaporating. Let the jar sit for at least 30-45 minutes or longer. The length of time and the amount of herbs you use will affect the strength of the tea.
(Step 4) Strain and serve.

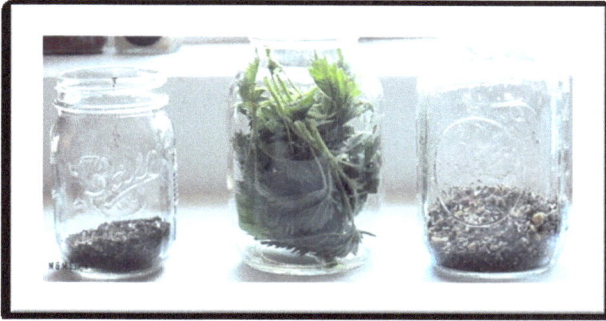

I personally like making my herbal infusions in the evening as it allows me to let them steep overnight so as to completely draw out the beneficial properties of the herbs.

7.   **DECOCTIONS** - Decoctions are preferred when the deep healing properties of roots, stems, and barks of plants are required. This process allows for the more tenacious plant constituents to be drawn out. This preparation is very similar to an infusion, but the herbs are simmered instead of steeped. Roots, rhizomes, some seeds, stems and barks are quite hard and their cell walls are very strong. In order to transfer the active constituents to the water, more heat is needed than when compared to infusions, and for that reason, the herb has to be boiled in water.

Instructions for Making an Herbal Decoction:

(Step 1) Place 1 ounce of herb(s) (chopped and bruised) into one pint of cold filtered or spring water.
(Step 2) With the heat on low, bring the mixture to a slow simmer for about 30 minutes.

95

(Step 3) Pour the mixture into a sterilized Mason jar and cover jar.

(Step 4) Set aside and let infuse overnight.

(Step 5) Strain and drink.

This should be used within 24 hours. For a stronger decoction, simmer for an additional 30 minutes.

8. **TINCTURES** - Tinctures are concentrated alcohol based extracts of plants that are quite potent and provide an effective way to administer herbal remedies. Tinctures are a great way to take herbs because they are so simple to make. You can make a relatively large amount with ease, and when stored properly in brown bottles, they last for several years, when compared to other herbal preparations. Tinctures are rather useful, especially when a chosen herb needs to be used over a long period. They are by far my favorite way of storing herbs. One ounce of tincture is equivalent to one ounce of herb.

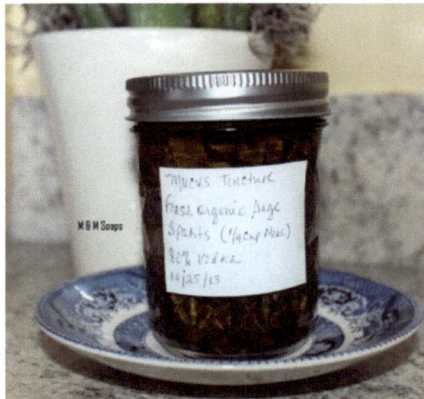

You have several options when choosing a solvent (i.e., liquid carrier) for your herbal tinctures: alcohol, food grade vegetable glycerin, water, or vinegar. If you use alcohol as your carrier, be sure to select one that is at least 80 to 100 proof. "Proof" relates to the actual alcohol/water content in the alcohol. For example, an 80-proof spirit is actually 40 percent alcohol and 40 percent water. A 100 proof spirit is 50 percent alcohol and 50 percent water. The ratio in the range of 50:50 (50 percent alcohol and 50 percent water) provides the perfect balance for extracting the most beneficial properties from herbs, which explains why most tinctured formulas you come across on the market today are typically made using an alcohol carrier. Most vodkas, gins, brandies, and rums available are 80 to 100 proof, so any one of them that is of high quality would work just fine in a tincture.

I personally prefer to use alcohol (Vodka) as a solvent because I believe it provides a more potent remedy. I find that the actual amount of alcohol you consume in any given remedy is negligible. Additionally, if you will be giving an alcohol based tinctured remedy to a small child, it is recommended that the alcohol be first completely evaporated before giving it to them. You do this by adding the indicated tincture drops to a glass with about 2 ounces of filtered water and waiting a few minutes before allowing the child to take the remedy.

If you prefer not to use alcohol at all due to conscientious reasons, you may use food grade vegetable glycerin or apple cider vinegar as a carrier instead. If you choose to make a tincture using vinegar, it is always best to use raw apple cider vinegar such as Braggs, as it will add even more health benefits to your tincture. Synthetic chemical vinegar should not be used. If you were to use raw cider vinegar as your carrier, you would follow the exact same instructions for the tincture as noted below.

Many herbalists like to put up their herbal tinctures at the exact time of the new moon and finish them off on the full moon, in order to take advantage of the natural drawing power attributed to the waxing moon.

If you use Glycerin as your carrier, you need to be sure to mix the amount of Glycerin (1:1 ratio) with one part water before adding it to the herbs. Glycerin based tinctures are sometimes preferred for children because they do not contain any traces of alcohol and they are generally milder on the digestive tract. Bear in mind however, that although they do work, non-alcohol tinctures are not as potent because these carriers are just not as effective at breaking down the plant constituents.

Instructions for Making an Herbal Tincture:

Never use rubbing alcohol, isopropyl alcohol, methyl, or wood alcohol for your tinctures – these are poisonous!

(Step 1) Place your selected and measured herb(s) in a large sterilized Mason jar (Refer to *Page 90* for the *Simpler's Measuring Method*).

(Step 2) Cover herbs completely with Vodka (or carrier of choice*). Stir herbs to make sure all of your ingredients are well incorporated.

(Step 3) Seal the jar tightly and give it a good shake.

(Step 4) Label your jar clearly (*Refer to Chapter 8, Par. 4*). Store your labeled jar in a cool dark place for at least 3 weeks.

(Step 5) Open jar and strain the herbs using cheesecloth.

(Step 6) Next, pour the liquid into a sterilized amber glass bottle.

(Step 7) Label the tincture bottle once again (Chap. 8, Par. 4).

*If you use Glycerin as your carrier, be sure to mix the amount of Glycerin (1:1 ratio) with one part water before adding it to the herbs.

Chapter 10
External Remedies

1.   **LINIMENTS**- Liniments are excellent remedy for relieving pain, aches, and muscular discomfort. They are typically used to stimulate and refresh the body, as they are an effective way to soothe sprains, muscle cramping, and strains. They can be used in the form of a massage, to relax the body, as well as to promote healing. Liniments can be made with an alcohol base or an oil base. I prefer to use rubbing alcohol in my liniments, as alcohol is a known rubefacient (which stimulates blood flow) and acts as a preservative for the remedy and gives it a longer shelf life.

If your Liniment is alcohol based, you should avoid applying it to the neck area, as rubbing alcohol in particular gives off powerful fumes. It is not harmful; however, some may be quite sensitive to the smell. If you must rub the chest area as in the case of congestion, I suggest you place a small towel loosely on the face of your subject, to lessen the

> After straining your herbal tea infusion, tincture, liniment, or decoction, do not throw away the spent herbs! Use them in your compost. Your garden will reward you for it!

effect of the fumes. Alcohol tends to evaporate quickly so you should keep the jar sealed and work relatively fast.

Instructions for Making an Herbal Liniment:

(Step 1) Place your selected and measured herbs in a clean Mason jar.
(Step 2) Pour approx. 16 ounces of Vodka or Rubbing Alcohol over the herbs and place the lid over the jar tightly.
(Step 3) Label the jar with a specific description of its contents and date.
(Step 4) Shake mixture up and place in a cool dark place for 7 days.
(Step 5) Strain the herbs from the liquid using cheesecloth. Work fast to avoid the evaporation of the alcohol.

> *Infusion vs. Decoction*:
> The process of steeping a plant in boiling water is called "infusion". The process of simmering a plant or its roots in lightly boiling water is called "decoction".

(Step 6) Place liquid back in clean jar and label the jar again. Also, be sure to mark the jar "For External Use Only". This is important, as you do not want anyone in your household confusing this with an internal remedy!

2.   **HERBAL MASSAGE OIL**- An herbal massage oil is a carrier oil that has been infused with herbs. Herbal massage oils are quite useful for external treatment of skin issues, for relaxing or soothing tired and sore muscles and for stimulating circulation throughout the body. When making herbal massage oils, my preferred base oils are olive and almond, because they have a relatively long shelf life and as a result, do not go rancid as quickly. Olive oil is also antimicrobial. The standard ratio is 1 ounce of herbs for 1 pint of carrier oil. I typically add a few drops of pure Vitamin E and/or Grapeseed Extract to the final product, as a natural preservative.

When making massage oils I would recommend that, you use dried herbs. Fresh herbs contain water and you do not want to introduce moisture into your oil, which can result in bacteria growth. Unless you are going to undergo the extra step of drying your fresh herbs in a dehydrator, oven,

> *When selecting a carrier for your herbal massage oil, choose Almond or Olive if you want oil that heals; choose Sesame, Sunflower, or Wheat Germ, if you want an oil that penetrates.*

or direct sun, before making your massage oil, it would be safer for you to use dried herbs.

Instructions for Making Herbal Massage Oil*:

(Step 1) Take 2 ounces of your selected herb(s) and place in a quart Mason jar.
 (Step 2) Add 1 pint of carrier oil to jar and seal with dry lid.
(Step 3) Place the jar directly in the sun for about two weeks. This will slowly extract the constituents and healing properties into the oil. If you do not want to wait two weeks, you may use the "bain marie" or water bath method, by taking a small pot and filling it with 3 cups of water. You want enough water in the pot to cover the outside of jar at least half way. Place your sealed jar with herbs inside this pot and place the pot in the oven. Turn on oven to 120°

for approximately 1 hour. After 1 hour, turn oven off and let the jar sit overnight.

(Step 4) Strain oil from herbs using cheesecloth.

(Step 5) Before placing oil back in clean jar, add about ¼ tspn of pure Vitamin E and/or Grapeseed Extract and any essential oils. The Vitamin E and/or Grapeseed Extract will help to extend the shelf life of the massage oil.

(Step 6) Label and store in a cool dry place.

(Note: If you are following the Herbal Massage Oil instructions as Step 1 to making the Herbal Salve, be sure to use the amount of oil indicated in the Salve formula).

*This same method may be utilized when preparing herbal oil infusions to use in the kitchen for your culinary endeavors.

3.   **HERBAL BATHS**- When most people take a bath, it is with the basic intention of getting clean. Nevertheless, there are many herbs which, when added to the water, can transform the bath experience into a soothing and healing water treatment. Imagine the benefits of immersing yourself in a strong infusion of herbal tea! An herbal bath can soften the skin, aid in circulation, relax the body, release accumulated toxins, and help heal skin issues. The effects of the herbs used intensify the longer you remain in the bath. The temperature of the bath helps to open up the pores and allows the herbal properties to be absorbed into your skin. Remember, you skin is your largest organ of elimination and assimilation. It is worth mentioning that both the water temperature and time spent in the tub play a critical role in how you will feel at the end of the bath.   If the temperature is too hot, you will feel drained and lethargic. If the water is too cold, it will not do enough to relieve the tension. You want the temperature to work with the herbs to regulate the body's circulation, reduce pain and any discomfort. The desired end result is that you come out of your bath feeling relaxed, calm and rejuvenated.

If you want a refreshing bath, stay in the tub for no longer than one hour and maintain the temperature between 92-95 degrees. If you are seeking more of a relaxing bath, consider no more than 15 to 30 minutes in the tub at 100 degrees. An herbal bath that is being administered for pain relief should be no longer than 10 minutes, with the water at 110 degrees. An herbal bath intended for relaxation would require at least ¼ cup of herbs. A therapeutic herbal bath would use at least 2 full ounces of herbs. Select your herbs based on what you want to accomplish: relaxation or healing, or both.

Instructions for Making an Herbal Bath:

(Step 1) Place your herbs (if intended for a relaxing bath ¼ cup, if for therapeutic purposes 2 ounces) in a stainless steel pot.
(Step 2) Add 1 quart of water, cover with lid, turn stove on, and allow it to simmer for about 10 minutes.
(Step 3) Turn off stove and let cool.
(Step 4) Strain with cheesecloth and add the liquid to your bath water.

4.   **SALVES** - Salves (or ointments) are quite easy to make and are very effective when dealing with skin conditions such as eczema, rashes, burns, boils, infections, bug bites, scrapes, splinters, and the like. Salves are made using a carrier oil, beeswax (vegans may opt to use carnauba or candelilla wax), and herbs. You may also choose to add pure essential oils in order to impart additional healing properties into your salves. They are also a simple way of nourishing and protecting the skin. I love the versatility salves provide and I strongly encourage you to make several varieties, using different herbal properties so that you have them at your disposal in your family's home emergency first aid kit.

The first step in making a salve involves making an oil infusion. A general rule of thumb when making salves is to use one part beeswax to four parts oil. If you are unhappy with the consistency of your finished salve, you can melt it again at low heat and adjust the ratios of wax to oil. More wax makes a more solid salve, while less wax gives the salve a creamier consistency. Bear in mind that in winter, you might prefer a creamier salve because room temperatures are generally cooler, while in summer, you might want a more solid salve (more wax) to compensate for warmer room temperatures. Feel free to experiment in order to arrive at a consistency that works for you.

Instructions for Making an Herbal Salve:

(Step 1) Take your selected and measured herb(s) and place in a quart Mason jar.

(Step 2) Add 2 ounces of your carrier oil (i.e., olive, almond, sunflower, sesame, etc.) and seal jar with a lid. Be sure that lid is completely dry to avoid getting any moisture into the jar.

(Step 3) Place the jar directly in the sun for about two weeks. This will slowly extract the constituents and healing properties into the oil. If you do not want to wait two weeks, you may use the "bain marie" or water bath method, by taking a small pot and filling it with 3 cups of water. You want enough water in the pot to cover the outside of jar at least half way. Place your sealed jar with herbs inside this pot and place the pot in the oven. Turn on oven to 120° for approximately 1 hour. After 1 hour, turn oven off and let the jar sit overnight.

(Step 4) Strain oil from herbs using cheesecloth.

(Step 5) Place your herbal infused oil back into a clean and dry glass jar and add your measured wax to the jar.

(Step 6) Using the "bain marie" or water bath method again, take a small pot and fill it with enough water to cover the outside of jar at least half way. Place your unsealed jar containing the infused oil and wax inside this pot, careful not to get any water inside the jar.

(Step 7) Turn stove on low heat (do not allow water to come to a boil as overheating will eliminate the beneficial healing properties of herbs and wax). Allow the wax to melt in very low heat. When the wax has completely melted you can do a quick consistency test by placing a spoon inside the mixture and allowing the spoon to cool off and solidify. This only takes a few minutes but it will save you the task of having to re-melt your salve in order to add more wax for a firmer result. If it is too soft, add a bit more wax; if you want a softer salve add more oil. Once it is at your desired consistency, you may remove it from heat and let sit for 2-3 minutes. Now you may add your essential oil, Vitamin E and/or Grapeseed Extract. Vitamin E and Grapeseed Extract will preserve and extend the salve's shelf life. Stir well with a chopstick or straw in order to incorporate well.

(Step 5) Carefully pour into tin or small glass jars.

(Step 6) Allow to harden (about one hour).

(Step 7) Label and store in a cool dry place where it will keep for several months.

Salves will melt if exposed to heat. Do not leave them in your car or exposed to direct sunlight. This will deteriorate the herbs and oil and make the salve go rancid quickly.

Chapter 11
Herbal Formulas

Herbal Bath

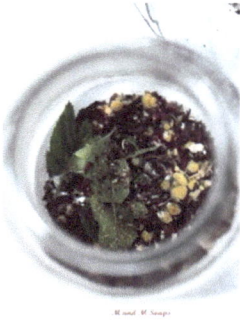

Tub baths are a commodity for me, so I thoroughly enjoy them on the rare occasion that I do have the opportunity to indulge in one. This relaxing herbal bath is a great way to end a long and stress filled day.

3 parts Lavender
2 Parts Peppermint
2 Parts Chamomile
2 Parts Basil
1 quart of water

Other Materials:
Stainless steel pot
Cheesecloth

Remember that the proportion of herbs indicated in this Herbal Bath recipe is for a relaxing bath. However, if you want to make this a therapeutic herbal bath you must increase the proportion of your herbs as noted in Page 101, to at least two full ounces.
Follow instructions on how to make Herbal Bath on Page 102

Other effective herbs to consider when making Herbal Baths:

Thyme, Sage, Comfrey, Marigold (Calendula), Elder

Winter Woes Capsules

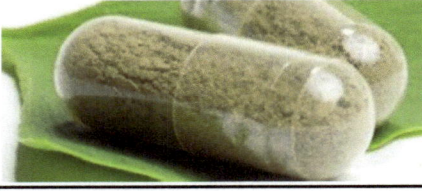

Keep these effective capsules handy for use at the first sign of a cold or flu. You will be amazed at how effective they are at boosting your immune system.

1 part Echinacea root powder
1 part Goldenseal root powder
½ part Marshmallow root powder
½-part Cayenne powder (could be less depending on your heat tolerance level)

Size "00" or "0" gelatin or vegetable capsules

Other materials:
Glass jar
 Label

Follow instructions for how to make Capsules on Page 92.
For usage, follow guidelines on Page 117.

Peppermint and Marigold (Calendula) Herbal Infusion

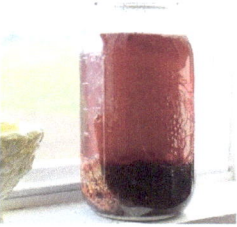

Enjoy this nourishing infusion during that time of the month, when experiencing menstrual pain, or anytime you need pampering.

1 Tbsp Marigold (Calendula)
1 Tbsp Peppermint
1 Tbsp Chamomile
1 Tbsp Red Raspberry
1 Tbsp Hibiscus flowers
1Tsp Stevia herb powder
2 quarts of filtered or spring water

Nettle is high in calcium, iron, protein, potassium, formic acid, beta-carotene, Vitamin K, and flavonoids.

Other Materials:
Sterilized Mason jar
Strainer

Please avoid this herbal infusion if you are pregnant

Follow instructions on how to make Herbal Infusion on Page 95. For usage, follow guidelines on Page 117.

Herbal Infusion for Healthy Skin

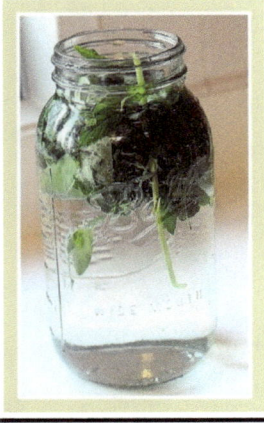

Try this infusion three times a day for several weeks to help clear up acne, eczema, psoriasis, blemishes or problem skin. It gently invigorates the liver and kidneys and allows it to remove accumulated waste, while the anti-inflammatory actions improve skin eruptions on the head, neck, and upper body. It also serves as a great detox infusion!

> **Tip:**
> *Drink 1-2 cups daily (use 1tsp of Milk Thistle <u>leaves</u>) when breastfeeding to stimulate milk production. For liver disorders drink 3 cups daily (use 1tsp of Milk Thistle <u>seeds</u>).*

2 Tbsp Dandelion
2 Tbsp Burdock leaf
2 Tbsp Red Clover
2 Tbsp Cleavers
1 Tsp Stevia herb powder
2 quarts of filtered or spring water

Other Materials:
Sterilized Mason jar
Strainer
Please avoid this herbal infusion if you are pregnant.
Follow instructions on how to make Herbal Infusion on Page 95.
For usage, follow guidelines on Page 117.

Herbal Liniment

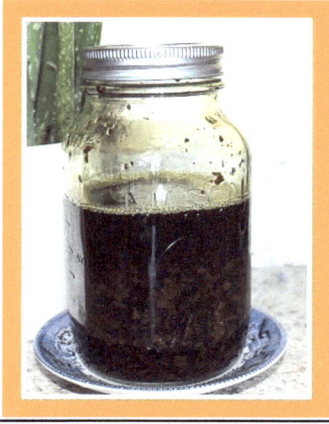

I have used this very effective Liniment on my husband whenever he experiences muscle and back pains. It provides him almost instant relief. Use it to soothe sprains, aches, muscle cramping, and strains.

Effective Combinations:

For depression, Oats may be used with Skullcap.

16 Oz Isopropyl Rubbing Alcohol (you may also use Vodka)
½ ounce Lobelia
1 ounce Eucalyptus
¼ ounce Cayenne
¼ ounce Ginger

Other Materials:
Sterilized quart Mason jar
Cheesecloth
Label (Please be sure to label your jar or bottle "**FOR EXTERNAL USE ONLY**!")

Follow instructions on how to make Liniment on Page 99.
For usage, follow guidelines on Page 117.

Other effective herbs to consider when making Liniments:

Wormwood, Golden Seal and Myrrh for fungus or skin issues.

Baby Herbal Massage Oil

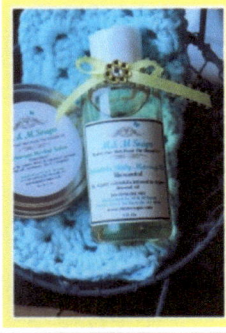

Human touch is essential to our well-being. I love Herbal Massage Oils because using them allows me the opportunity to stay connected with my little ones. We enjoy them after a bath and before bedtime. This allows me to bond with them, talk to them about the day's events, and find out what is on their minds. In doing this, I am also showing them by example how to stay in touch with their bodies. Massaging them regularly allows me to notice any abnormality, bug bite, scratch, bump, etc., which might not have otherwise been noticed.

Mullein flower oil is an effective treatment for ear infections that are caused by upper respiratory congestion. A few warm drops on each ear relieve pain within minutes and reverses infection within a few days.

2 parts Marigold (Calendula)
2 parts Chamomile
3 ounces Almond oil
Vitamin E and Grapeseed Extract
 Essential Oils (optional)

Other Materials:
3 to 4 Oz bottle
Cheesecloth
Label
Follow instructions on how to make Herbal Massage Oil on Page 100.

Hyssop Oxymel

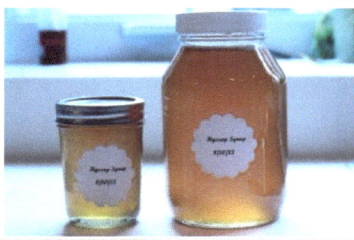

I always keep this easy to make Oxymel in our cupboard for use at the beginning of the winter season, in order to boost everyone's immunity and ward off colds. The children absolutely love it!

Hyssop (enough to fill quart size jar ½ way)
Raw honey (enough to fill jar 1/3 way)
Raw apple cider vinegar (enough to fill jar)

Other Materials:

Sterilized quart size Mason jar
Strainer
Labels

Pregnant women should not take Hyssop.

Follow instructions for how to make Oxymels on Page 91.
For usage, follow guidelines on Page 117.

Other effective herbs to consider when making Oxymels and Syrups that target upper respiratory infections are: Thyme and Oregano (both are anti-viral and anti-bacterial).

Plantain and Marigold (Calendula) Salve

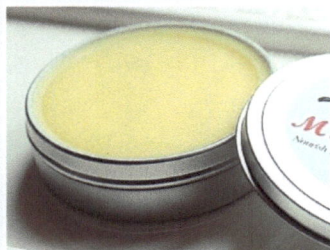

This salve is part of our natural first aid kit. Plantain is known for its antihistamine action and Marigold (Calendula) is known for its antiseptic and healing properties. We use this salve for rashes, insect bites, scrapes, cuts, and abrasions.

1 Tbsp Plantain leaf
1 Tbsp Marigold (Calendula)
3 ounces Olive oil (for oil infusion)
2 Tbsp beeswax
Vitamin E and Grapeseed Extract
 Essential Oils (optional)

Other Materials:
Metal tin or small jar container
Cheesecloth
Label

Effective combinations:

For stomach issues Goldenseal combines well with Chamomile. Externally as a wash for irritation and itching, it works well with distilled Witch Hazel. Can be combined with Mullein and used as ear drops.

Follow instructions for how to make Salve on Pages 103. For usage, follow guidelines on Page 117.

Refreshing Herbal Tea

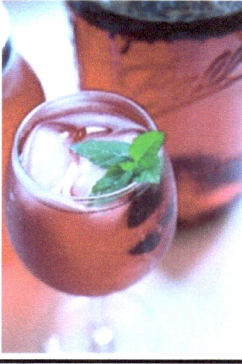

Curb your family's craving for sugary drinks with this refreshing Herbal Tea. This is one of my family's favorite herbal combinations. It is kid approved!

1 Tbsp Chamomile
1 Tbsp Peppermint
1 Tbsp Lemon balm
1 Tbsp Hibiscus flowers
1Tsp Stevia herb powder
2 quarts of filtered or spring water

Other Materials:
Sterilized Mason jar
Strainer

Effective Combinations:

For colds and fevers, combine Elder with Peppermint, Yarrow, or Hyssop.

Follow instructions on how to make Herbal Tea on Page 94.
For usage, follow guidelines on Page 117.

Deep Sleep Herbal Tincture

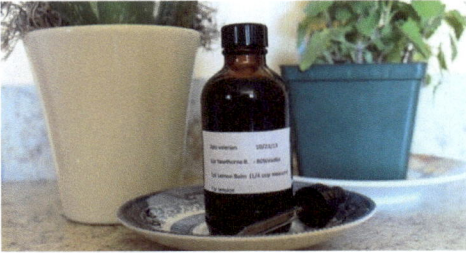

This is a gentle non-habit forming tincture, which will help you get a good night's sleep. I receive many requests for this tincture from family and friends. It is quite effective!

1 part Valerian Root
1 part Hops
½ part Lavender
80 or 100 proof Vodka

Other Materials:
Sterilized Mason jar
Cheesecloth
Label

Effective Combinations:

For microbial infections, Garlic will combine well with Echinacea.

Follow instructions on how to make Tincture on Page 98 and refer to Simpler's Measuring Method on Page 90.

For usage, follow guidelines on Page 117.

Calendula (Marigold) Tincture

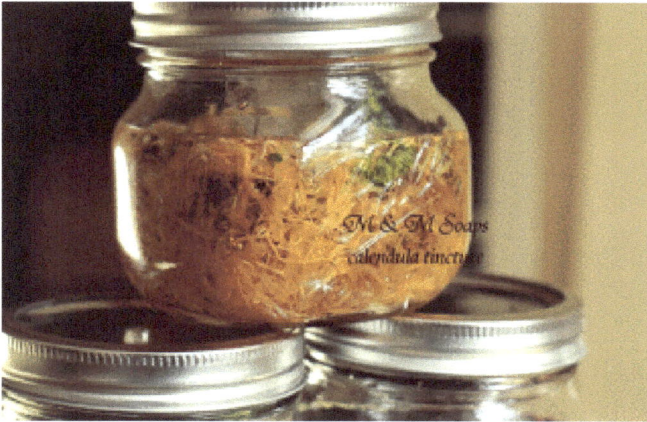

I use this formula for moon cycle discomfort, and so much more. You can use it as a go to remedy whenever calendula is indicated (i.e., for burns, fungus infections, bruises, nosebleeds, itching).

2 parts Calendula (Marigold)
80 or 100 proof Vodka

Other Materials:
Sterilized Mason jar
Cheesecloth
Label

Effective combinations:

To assist in stopping heavy menstrual bleeding, use Plantain with Yarrow and Nettle.

Follow instructions on how to make Tincture on Page 98 and refer to Simpler's Measuring Method on Page 90.

For usage, follow guidelines on Page 117.

Elderberry Tincture

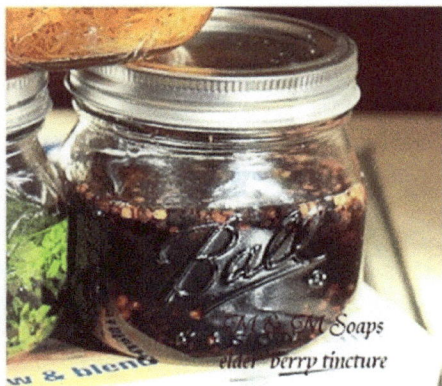

No household should be without Elderberry tincture. This is a simple, no fuss formula that is quite effective in boosting everyone's immunity prior to and during the cold winter season. This tincture is also an excellent source of Potassium.

Effective combinations:

For gastric problems, Licorice may be combined with Marshmallow and Comfrey.

2 parts Elder berries
80 or 100 proof Vodka

Other Materials:
Sterilized Mason jar
Cheesecloth
Label

Follow instructions on how to make Tincture on Page 98 and refer to Simpler's Measuring Method on Page 90.

For usage, follow guidelines on Page 117.

Chapter 12
Dosage and Other Considerations

It is very difficult to give an exact dosage to be followed in every case, as each person has a different body, temperament, etc. and naturally, all of this will play a role in how one responds to any given remedy. The general rule adhered to by master herbalists is to begin with the smallest dose first and work toward gradually larger doses, if needed. The dose is also to be altered depending on the age of the individual. For example, a ten year-old child usually will require half the adult dose; a five year-old child can generally be given one-quarter of an adult dose.

Dosage for Acute Issues:
½ to 1 Tsp of herbal syrup every 2 hours, up to 10 Tsp daily
¼ to ½ Tsp of herbal tincture every hour, up to 6 Tsp daily
One herbal capsule or pill every 2 hours, up to 8 capsules daily

Dosage for Chronic Illness:
3 to 4 cups of herbal tea daily
1 to 2 Tbsp of herbal syrup twice daily or as needed
½ to 1 Tsp of tincture 2 or 3 times daily, up to 3 Tsp daily
2 or 3 capsules or pills 2 or 3 times daily, up to 6 capsules

As mentioned above, an individual's temperament will affect how the remedy is received. Therefore, it is wise to give nervous, high-strung persons smaller and more frequent doses.

In addition, when applying diuretics, it is better to begin with small doses, so that the kidneys are not over-worked when in a weakened condition.

Capsules

Dosage in capsules is completely dependent upon the age, sex, general health, and nature of the condition. A general rule is to give capsules (by capsule size) as follows:

Capsule #0 (holds 475mg): 3, three times per day, with meals.
Capsule #00 (holds 665mg): 2, three times per day.
Capsule # 4 (holds 145mg): 1, five or six times per day.

Capsule #2 (holds 260mg): 2 upon waking up, two at bedtime.

Infusions

One cup three times per day is the general rule, although there is great variation in dosage of infusions.

Liniments

Always do a patch test in the forearm before applying Liniments. Rub or massage the Liniment onto the affected area making sure it is all absorbed into the skin. Work fast so as to avoid allowing all of the alcohol to evaporate. Cover up your subject with a towel after applying the Liniment to the desired area(s). This will allow the herbs to generate a warming sensation. Apply as often as needed.

Oxymels

One mouthful as a gargle, or as directed.

Salves

Use enough to cover the area, but not so much that residue is left on the skin.

Syrups

According to size and age: 1 teaspoon to 1 tablespoon.

Tinctures

One ounce of tincture is equal in strength to approximately 1 ounce of the powdered herb, so 3 drops will be equal to 1/2 cup of tea. For children or those sensitive to alcohol, always dilute tincture dosage in 1 to 2 ounces of filtered water and let sit for at least two minutes in order to allow the alcohol to evaporate before drinking.

Chapter 13
Reading Recommendations

I strongly recommend that you acquire at least one good reference book for furthering your herbal knowledge. There is so much more for you to learn about these amazing plants, beyond what I have shared with you here. A good herbal reference will be invaluable to you on this journey. There are many books available online and at your local library. I personally have been successful in finding quite a few excellent herbal books at our local thrift store.

Once you start experimenting with this beautiful art of healing and you start experiencing results, you may discover that this is your true calling and you may be moved to expand your knowledge beyond the resources being shared in this book. I wholeheartedly encourage you to do so and as you learn, pay it forward. That is, continue to pass on your newfound knowledge and love of herbs, so that the life of others may also be enriched in the process. If we each strive to do this, we allow ourselves to be used as a tool to effect the larger scale change we want our children and their future generations to experience.

Some of my favorite herbal reference books are:

Healing Wise, by Susun S. Weed

The Secret Life of Plants, by Peter Tompkins

Practical Herbalism, by Philip Fritchey

The Complete Medicinal Herbal: A Practical Guide to the Healing Properties of Herbs, by Penelope Ody

Wise Woman Herbal for the Childbearing Year, by Susun S. Weed

Chapter 14
Resources and References

Below you will find websites and links that might prove helpful to you when sourcing herbs, jars to store your remedies, as well as educational links pertaining to wellness and nutrition. Although these online sources are provided, I encourage you to buy local, whenever and as often as possible.

1. Packaging for your Remedies

   Sourcing brown bottles to store remedies:
   Abundant Health
   http://www.abundanthealth4u.com/

   Sourcing capsule filler machine:
   Apple Tree Bulk Herbs
   http://www.appletreebulkherbs.ca/capsules-for-herbs.php

2. Educational & Nutritional Resources

   Weston A. Price Foundation (Traditional Foods Educational Site)
   http://www.westonaprice.org/

   Cultures for Health (Kombucha & Yogurt Cultures & Kefir Grains)
   http://www.culturesforhealth.com/

3. Herb Seeds for your Garden

   Annie's Heirloom Seeds
   27300 Sloptown Road
   Beaver Island, MI 4982

4. High Quality Dried Herbs

   Mountain Rose Herbs* (Affiliate)
   https://www.mountainroseherbs.com/?AID=133790&BID=13910

Monterey Bay spice Co.
http://www.herbco.com/

5. Local Farm Foods

Source local dairy, meats, honey, vegetables, etc. where you live:
http://www.localharvest.org/

6. Artisan handcrafted bath and body products, formulated with herbs, natural colorants, pure essential oils and wholesome ingredients:

MMSoaps
http://www.mnmsoaps.com

7. Herbal Contraindications

http://www.holisticonline.com/Herbal-Med/hol_herb_med_reac.htm

8. Natural Feminine Hygiene – Cloth Pads

Root Woman Earth Child
http://www.etsy.com/shop/rootwomanearthchild

9. Portable Water Filer

Berkey Water Filters
http://www.berkeyfilters.com

Chapter 15
Herbs and Their Nutritional Value

Vitamins are essential elements for our health and for the normal function of our body systems. Herbs and plants can provide us with a full variety of vitamins, which are necessary for our wellbeing. Natural minerals such as magnesium, selenium, calcium, iron, and manganese are very common and can be found in many medicinal herbs. At the same time, such minerals like copper, iodine, sulfur and phosphorus are considered rare, but they are also needed by our body to support life. By using medicinal herbs and plants as a source for these vitamins and minerals, we receive from Mother Nature the support we need to nourish our body.

Vitamin A:

Alfalfa, Basil, Cayenne, Comfrey, Dandelion, Elderberries, Nettles, Parsley, Paprika, Raspberry leaf, Lamb's Quarters, Watercress Yellow Dock, Peppermint, Rosemary, Sage

Vitamin B Complex:

Comfrey, Red Clover, Parsley, Garlic, Peppermint, Sage, Turmeric

Thiamine, Vitamin B1:

Dandelion, Alfalfa, Red Clover, Fenugreek, Parsley, Raspberry leaf, Seaweeds such as Nori and Kelp, Catnip

Riboflavin, Vitamin B2:

Rose hips, Parsley, Dandelion, Dulse, Kelp, Fenugreek

Pyridoxine, Vitamin B12:

Alfalfa, Comfrey, Seaweeds such as Dulse and Kelp, Catnip

Niacin, Vitamin B Factor:

Burdock root and seed, Dandelion, Alfalfa, Parsley, Borage

Vitamin C:

Elderberries, Rose hips, Parsley, Cayenne, Dandelion greens, Red Clover, Burdock, Comfrey, Plantain, Nettles, Wormwood, Alfalfa, Borage, Garlic, Peppermint, Rosemary, Sage, Turmeric

Vitamin D:

Alfalfa, Nettles

Vitamin E:

Alfalfa, Rose hips, Raspberry leaf, Dandelion, Seaweeds such as Nori and Kelp, Borage, Burdock, Turmeric

Vitamin K:

Alfalfa, Nettles, Kelp, Basil, Dandelion, Parsley

Calcium:

Alfalfa, Red Clover, Raspberry leaf, Comfrey, Nettles, Parsley, Cleavers, Horsetail, Plantain, Chamomile, Shepherd's Purse, Borage, Dandelion, Kelp, Dulse, Thyme, Burdock, Garlic, Peppermint, Rosemary, Sage, Turmeric

Copper:

Alfalfa, Parsley, Nettles, Borage, Garlic, Ginger, Peppermint, Rosemary, Sage, Turmeric

Fluorine:

Garlic

Iodine:

Parsley, Sarsaparilla, Seaweeds such as Kelp and Dulse

Iron:

Nettles, Dandelion, Alfalfa, Yellow Dock, Chickweed, Burdock, Kelp, Mullein, Parsley, Comfrey, Fennel, Thyme, Borage, Garlic, Peppermint, Rosemary, Sage, Turmeric

Magnesium:

Alfalfa, Parsley, Mullein, Dulse, Dandelion greens, Burdock, Ginger, Peppermint, Rosemary, Sage, Turmeric

Manganese:

Alfalfa, Parsley, Thyme, Burdock, Dandelion, Garlic, Ginger, Peppermint, Rosemary, Sage, Turmeric

Phosphorus:

Parsley, Nettles, Chickweed, Alfalfa, Licorice, Marigold petals, Raspberry leaf, Dandelion, Comfrey

Potassium:

Chamomile, Comfrey, Nettles, Dandelion, Alfalfa, Yarrow, Borage, Peppermint, Plantain, Parsley, Kelp, Dulse, Thyme, Ginger, Rosemary, Sage, Turmeric

Silicon:

Horsetail, Dandelion, Nettles

Sulphur:

Nettles, Plantain, Parsley, Garlic, Mullein, Shepherd's Purse, Sage